MW00770835

# Pennhurst and the Struggle for Disability Rights

*Edited by*

Dennis B. Downey
and James W. Conroy

*With a foreword by*

DICK AND GINNY THORNBURGH

The Pennsylvania State University Press
University Park, Pennsylvania

**KEYSTONE BOOKS**

Keystone Books are intended to serve the citizens of Pennsylvania. They are accessible, well-researched explorations into the history, culture, society, and environment of the Keystone State as part of the Middle Atlantic region.

Library of Congress Cataloging-in-Publication Data

Names: Downey, Dennis B., 1952– editor. | Conroy, James W., 1948– editor.
Title: Pennhurst and the struggle for disability rights / edited by Dennis B. Downey and James W. Conroy ; with a foreword by Dick and Ginny Thornburgh.
Description: University Park, Pennsylvania : The Pennsylvania State University Press, [2020] | "Keystone books." | Includes bibliographical references and index.
Summary: "A comprehensive study of the history of the Pennhurst State School and Hospital (1908–87), a state-operated institution in Pennsylvania for children and adults with intellectual and developmental disabilities. Explores Pennhurst's enduring impact on the disability civil rights movement in America"—Provided by publisher.
Identifiers: LCCN 2019059655 | ISBN 9780271086033 (cloth)
Subjects: LCSH: Pennhurst State School (Pa.)—History. | Intellectual disability facilities patients—Care—Pennsylvania—History—20th century. | Intellectual disability facilities patients—Abuse of—Pennsylvania—History—20th century. | Intellectual disability facilities patients—Deinstitutionalization—Pennsylvania—History—20th century. | Intellectual disability facilities patients—Legal status, laws, etc.—Pennsylvania—History—20th century.
Classification: LCC HV3006.P42 P45 2020 | DDC 362.2/10974813—dc23
LC record available at https://lccn.loc.gov/2019059655


Printed in the United States of America
Published by The Pennsylvania State University Press,
University Park, PA 16802–1003

The Pennsylvania State University Press is a member of the Association of University Presses.

It is the policy of The Pennsylvania State University Press to use acid-free paper. Publications on uncoated stock satisfy the minimum requirements of American National Standard for Information Sciences—Permanence of Paper for Printed Library Material, ANSI Z39.48–1992.

To the lives, memory, and lasting contribution of the 10,600 people who lived at Pennhurst during its seventy-nine-year history. They represent the lives of approximately six hundred thousand American citizens with intellectual and developmental disabilities who lived in public institutions from 1850 to the present. Their struggles and their triumphs have helped change the nation's policies.

## *Contents*

# *Illustrations*

## GALLERIES (FOLLOWING PAGE 233)

## FIGURES



## TABLES

## *Foreword*

DICK AND GINNY THORNBURGH

The story of Pennhurst is central to an understanding of the disability civil rights movement in America. The legal and ethical implications of the issues surrounding that institution shaped much of our own thinking about Americans with disabilities while we were in the Governor's Residence in Pennsylvania—and forever thereafter. We are pleased and honored to be asked to introduce this volume of historic writings about the multiple meanings of Pennhurst in our history.

In the late 1960s and early 1970s, Ginny was a volunteer with the Allegheny County Chapter Pennsylvania Arc. Ginny and Dick's third son, Peter Thornburgh, had both intellectual and physical disabilities, and it was this organization that taught her how to fight for his rights. Although Peter lived at home with his parents and three brothers, Ginny became interested in those children and adults with developmental and intellectual disabilities who were not able to live at home. She and a small group of well-trained volunteers visited nearly all of Pennsylvania's state schools and hospitals and numerous interim care facilities. Many of these visits were unannounced and revealed shocking conditions.

As the governor of Pennsylvania from 1979 to 1987, Dick was charged with the daunting duty of seeking justice in the complex litigation concerning Pennhurst State School and Hospital—a facility that had been operating since 1908 to house Pennsylvanians with developmental and intellectual disabilities. By 1979, there were nearly eight thousand citizens with developmental and intellectual disabilities in Pennsylvania's large public institutions—Pennhurst was just one of twelve. In the words of Bill Baldini, in a follow-up to his original

1968 exposé of conditions at Pennhurst, these eight thousand children and adults were "no less precious" than any other Pennsylvanians. We knew that resolving the issue of Pennhurst in the courts would affect countless others.

By the time Dick took office, the major courtroom drama had been completed. The prior state administration had fought hard to keep the federal court from demanding Pennsylvania change the way it supported people at places like Pennhurst. But on March 17, 1978, Federal District Court Judge Raymond Broderick issued an extraordinary and unprecedented order. Because the parties were unable to reach an amicable settlement, Judge Broderick decided to order Pennsylvania to provide small homes in regular neighborhoods with full 24-hour supervision and assistance for every person at Pennhurst.

Privately, we applauded this decision and order. Never before had a federal court acted with such courage on behalf of people who had been hidden away, ignored by the media and the citizens, and subjected to routine underfunding, understaffing, segregation, and all too often, abuse and neglect of dimensions unbelievable to most Americans.

An immediate search was initiated by the Thornburgh administration for a new deputy secretary of the Department of Public Welfare, for the Office of Mental Retardation (that was the terminology in those days). By far the best-qualified and most capable candidate was Dr. Jennifer Howse, who negotiated with the governor's office with unshakeable integrity. Her firm condition for accepting the job was to be permitted a free hand in the careful, proper, and life-affirming reintegration of the folks at Pennhurst into the mainstream of community life. We were delighted to "cave in" to this demand!

Over the next eight years, Dr. Howse worked unceasingly to secure our commitment to provide mainstream living to all the residents of our "Pennhursts" in Pennsylvania. A signal accomplishment in this effort occurred during Dick's last year in office when the amount of state funding sought for community facilities finally exceeded the amount allocated to institutional living. It was then that we figuratively "broke out the champagne of celebration"!

Nevertheless, despite continuing litigation and appeals because of issues not actually related to justice and the integration of folks with disabilities—that, of course, was a settled issue—Pennsylvania began the hard work of providing new lives in the community for all.

By January of 1987, Dick had finished his two terms as the governor of the Commonwealth. In November of that year, the last two gentlemen moved from their large hospital-like "cottage" or "ward" at Pennhurst into their new community homes. The process of the closure, under the leadership of Dr. Howse and the courage and strong advocacy of the Arc of Pennsylvania and thousands of others who made the process work, formed a body of work well worth close and careful examination.

We now know, from the remarkable improvements in qualities of life as documented by the Pennhurst Longitudinal Study, that this transition from institution to community was one of the most successful social changes of the past half century. The Pennhurst accomplishments stand in stark contrast to the nation's dismal record of deinstitutionalization in the mental health field. In the case of people with developmental and intellectual disabilities, community placement was done with care and caution—to ensure that no one moved until all their supports were in place in their new community home.

The story of this remarkable revolution and the monumental place where it unfolded has never been fully told. Consequently, and perhaps also as a result of this oversight, the accomplishments achieved are also not fully understood. We are sure that American advocates, citizens, and scholars, as well as peers in other countries, will benefit from the story that is finally fully told in this book.

# Acknowledgments

Writing or editing a book is not a solitary effort, especially when there are so many contributors with varied backgrounds and expertise. For the editors, this has been a blissful yet daunting collaboration. Like the editors and principal authors, each of the contributors shares a commitment to telling the Pennhurst story in all of its complexity, and advancing a scholarly and social awareness of the disability civil rights struggle. Despite quite different perspectives, the contributors to this volume share the belief that there is more to Pennhurst than Pennhurst. History is something that happens to people, and the legacy of tragedy and triumph—memory and hope—embedded in this narrative speaks to the meaning of history and the human condition.

We are indebted to the people who lived the reality of the Pennhurst saga. A half century after Pennhurst's closing, it is impossible to fully appreciate the courage and resilience required to place a family's name on the original lawsuit list—the "named plaintiffs" in *Halderman v. Pennhurst*. We hereby salute and thank them:

TERRI LEE HALDERMAN, by her mother and guardian, Winifred Halderman;

LARRY TAYLOR, by his parents and guardians, Elmer and Doris Taylor;

KENNY TAYLOR, a minor, by his parents and guardians, Elmer and Doris Taylor;

ROBERT SOBETSKY, a minor, by his parents and guardians, Frank and Angela Sobetsky;

THERESA SOBETSKY, by her parents and guardians, Frank and Angela Sobetsky;

NANCY BETH BOWMAN, by her parents and guardians, Mr. and Ms. Horace Bowman;

LINDA TAUB, by her parents and guardians, Mr. and Ms. Allen Taub;
GEORGE SOROTOS, a minor, by his foster parents, William and Marion Caranfa;
THE PARENTS AND FAMILY ASSOCIATION OF PENNHURST

Many individuals and organizations have assisted in the research and preparation of this manuscript. We thank our contributors, research archivists, librarians, and disability rights advocates, who have shared their knowledge and expertise, and in some cases their personal stories. The Public Interest Law Center of Philadelphia hosted a meeting where this project was first conceived. Special mention must be given to the National Archives, the Pennsylvania State Archives and Library, the City of Philadelphia Archives, the American Philosophical Society, and the Library of the Philadelphia College of Physicians. Beth Lander and the library staff were exceptionally helpful in facilitating research and answering questions. We are grateful to the members of the Board of Directors of the Pennhurst Memorial and Preservation Alliance, and the Commissioners of the Pennsylvania Historical and Museum Commission. Kathleen Pavelko, Cara Williams Fry, and Keira McGuire at WITF Media, Inc., have been instrumental in documenting the history of intellectual disability in Pennsylvania and bringing that knowledge to a wide audience. Radio Smart Talk host Scott Lamar interviewed us several times.

Thomas and Gillian Gilhool, Senator Robert Casey and his staff, and especially disability policy aide Dr. Michael Gamel-McCormick, have encouraged this project in numerous ways. Tom and Gillian have provided an example of courageous and creative engagement in the struggle for disability rights, which is, after all, the struggle for human rights. Millersville University and Provost Vilas Prabhu, PhD, provided financial assistance and a sabbatical leave. On numerous occasions Barbara Erdman and Maggie Eichler, and a cohort of students in the University Honors College, assisted with logistics and with conference support.

Among the many presentations that grew out of this research, TASH International, the Pennsylvania Historical Association, Millersville University, and the National Constitution Center were gracious hosts. Charlene Mires, Tamara Gaskell, and the staff of the Mid-Atlantic Regional Center for the Humanities sponsored a lively session at the Rutgers-Camden Conference Center. In November 2017, The Historical Society of Pennsylvania convened an important symposium on Pennhurst and the history of disabilities, attracting nearly two hundred participants. A capacity crowd attended a session devoted to Pennhurst at the 2018 Mid-Atlantic Regional Archives Conference (MARAC).

This book would not have been completed without the generous encouragement and kind persistence of Kathryn B. Yahner, Laura Reed-Morrison, Hannah N. Hebert, and the editorial staff at Penn State University Press. Kathryn in particular has been the model editor and advocate for this manuscript. We are grateful for her patience and wise counsel. Dana Henricks was a precise and considerate copy-editor who improved the manuscript in numerous ways. Dr. Susan Ortmann skillfully prepared the index. We thank the anonymous reviewers who critiqued an earlier version of this manuscript and made cogent recommendations.

In that regard, Dr. Charles Hardy III of West Chester University has been a critical reader in the best sense of the word. His occasional queries—"How's the book, are you finished?"—served as a necessary prompt to keep at it. Similarly, Dr. Francis Bremer, Clarence Maxwell, Saulius Sužiedėlis, and John Osborne listened patiently and offered sound feedback. Dr. Donald Yacovone of Harvard's Huggins Institute has been an invaluable sounding board on all things historical. As is his way, Dr. Randall Miller has been unfailingly kind and encouraging in affirming the significance of Pennhurst and the necessity to tell this story.

The Temple University Developmental Disabilities Center, now the Institute on Disabilities, offered a unique vantage point from which to watch the Pennhurst saga unfold. Many families, experts, leaders, and researchers found a platform through which a permanent record of the victories could be crafted. First among the professional who make this work possible was the director, Dr. Edward Newman. He supervised the activation of Section 504 of the Rehabilitation Act—the disability civil rights law—while in Washington, and then offered

Temple University as a safe haven for free intellectual inquiry as state misdeeds unfolded. His moral courage in the face of political pressures cannot be overstated. Other Temple personnel deserving some recognition include Professor of Statistics John Flueck and Center coworkers Philip Jones, Jim Lemanowicz, Celia Feinstein, Scott Spreat, Hoyt Walbridge, Ken Thurman, and Dan Keating. Now-deceased allies Thom Cramer, Mike McAllister, and Bob Walsh deserve recognition as well.

Finally, Dennis Downey wishes to thank his wife Traci and each of his children—Bernie, Maggie, Kara, Thomas, and Anna—for once again enduring the vagaries of a distracted historian. Words are powerful but fail to capture the enormous gift of love and meaning they give to my life. To each, and especially to Traci, I thank them for being themselves and for helping me find my true self.

Jim Conroy's family offered him continuous encouragement and patience. In his words, "My immediate and loving family are always in my thoughts of gratitude: parents Al and Sis, wife Irene, kids Nora and Nicholas, brothers and sisters Tom, Dick, and Marianne, and cousins Janet and Amos."

# Introduction

DENNIS B. DOWNEY AND JAMES W. CONROY

On April 10, 2010, nearly three hundred people gathered along a roadside outside Spring City in Chester County, Pennsylvania. Of diverse backgrounds, abilities, and life experiences, they assembled to dedicate a historical marker to commemorate the Pennhurst State School and Hospital and its importance to the disability rights movement. The Pennhurst Memorial and Preservation Alliance (PMPA) and the Public Interest Law Center of Philadelphia (PILCOP) were the chief advocates for a state marker, based on a proposal first offered by attorney Thomas K. Gilhool. Two years in the planning, this simple seventy-word marker acknowledged more than a century of historical significance and ongoing public controversy surrounding Pennhurst. Dozens of community organizations with some affiliation with disability policy joined the campaign.

Originally licensed (1903) as the Eastern Pennsylvania State Institution for the Feeble-Minded and Epileptic, Pennhurst doubled in size to a cottage-style campus of more than 1,200 acres including 125 acres of buildings and grounds. Conceived for no more than 500 residents when it opened in 1908, in its heyday more than 3,500 residents lived on the grounds, supported by a staff of six hundred. In all, more than 10,600 residents occupied Pennhurst during its eight decades of operation (1908–87).[1] Male and female, black and white, and of varying abilities and often confused and incorrect diagnoses, the residents led segregated lives within a custodial environment far removed from the social mainstream. Those who could work toiled at menial jobs in the shops and fields, or janitorial care to support the institution. It was an arrangement not unlike peonage or servile labor, meant to maximize profitability. All the residents were said to have some degree of congenital mental "defect," or in today's parlance an intellectual disability.

In a particular sense, the historical marker was an attempt to come to terms with history, and the history of a particular place and its residents. For some this marker was a public acknowledgment of Pennhurst's freighted legacy of exploitation and abuse, and to others it was a sign of hope for a different future. Furthermore, the day served as a reminder that history is a lived experience, and that history is something that happens to people. Eight years later, this metallic sign still stands as an act of remembrance, just feet from the now overgrown lane that leads through woods to the long-abandoned Pennhurst campus along the Schuylkill River. (Most of the buildings have been demolished to make way for a commercial park; the ever-popular "Pennhurst Asylum" venue that draws tens of thousands of paying customers each Halloween season remains intact.)

The day's speakers included elected officials, attorneys, advocates, and self-advocates who had championed the cause of individuals with disabilities in the courts, in the halls of government, and in the court of public opinion. Betty Potts, the first resident to leave Pennhurst under a federal court order in 1978, was on hand, as was former resident Nicholas Romeo. So too was Jean Searle, once institutionalized herself and now copresident of the Pennhurst Memorial and Preservation Alliance. Like many of the attendees, all three were part of the sea change in public policy that established the ability of people to live less segregated and stigmatized lives through deinstitutionalization. Many remembered Roland Johnson, another person who had emerged from Pennhurst to tell the story of his role in self-advocacy for equal rights. In a similar vein, participants were reminded of the important roles Terri Lee Halderman and Nicholas Romeo played in groundbreaking litigation over conditions at Pennhurst.[2]

Attorneys Thomas Gilhool and Judith Gran shared recollections, as did Dennis Haggerty, Pat Clapp, and newsman Bill Baldini. Nathaniel Guest, who had taken an interest in the history of Pennhurst as a teenager and later helped to found the PMPA, presided over the dedication itself. An entire generation of private nonprofit service providers had come into being to support the Pennhurst exodus, and many of those deeply committed public servants were in attendance. For many the dedication day was a kind of homecoming, or a reunion in a common cause they had fought for more than forty years.

By 1923, the Commonwealth of Pennsylvania was providing complete or partial financial support to more than sixty facilities that cared for individuals with some diagnosed mental illness, disability, or debilitating medical condition.[3] A companion facility to Polk State School and Hospital in western Pennsylvania (and a state-supported private training school at Elwyn), Pennhurst was tied intimately to public health circles in Philadelphia, and the city's great medical colleges. Conceived, financed, and sustained by state government appropriations, Pennhurst was a creature of Pennsylvania and national public health concerns over the rising tide of what some medical professionals and their political allies viewed as "enfeebled" and "degenerate" fellow citizens—mental and moral *defectives*, some said—best separated from the general population and the gene pool.[4]

Once thought of as a model state institution for the training and care of individuals with intellectual and developmental disabilities, Pennhurst was shuttered in 1987 and the residents relocated following a series of jarring news reports that revealed a pattern of neglect, mistreatment, and dehumanizing conditions, and a federal consent decree that resulted from a decade of litigation. In truth, however, decades of political advocacy and court arguments paved the way for Pennhurst's closing. Three groundbreaking court cases—*PARC v. Commonwealth of Pennsylvania*; *Halderman v. Pennhurst State School and Hospital* (Halderman v. Pennhurst State School and Hospital, 446 F. Supp. 1295) and *Romeo v. Youngberg*—are now considered to be landmark decisions in American jurisprudence.[5]

Like hundreds of institutions across the United States and parts of Europe, places with names like Vineland, Willowbrook, Polk and Forest Haven, Sonoma State, and Jacksonville, Pennhurst was a testament to modern scientific and social engineering at the dawn of the American Century. The champions of institutionalization were as often animated by eugenics and the so-called "science of better breeding" as they were diagnostic and clinical reforms. Its creators and their political allies imagined Pennhurst as an icon to "progress" and "improvement" in the care of individuals with "hereditary feeble-mindedness" and other debilitating mental conditions. Guardians of the future and the public good, or so they thought, eugenicists embraced the language and activism of public stigma to further marginalize the most vulnerable members of society. Mass institutionalization went hand in hand with the growing professionalization of medical science and eugenic social thought.

Buoyed by a burgeoning national public health movement, new techniques for behavioral therapy, and the invention of new diagnostic terminology, the architects of institutionalization included some of most enlightened cultural and medical minds of the age. By the close of the nineteenth century, these forces had converged in Pennsylvania and elsewhere to exert tremendous influence on public policy. Institutionalization of those said to be hereditarily "defective" was a global phenomenon, most notable in the United States and Europe, and in Japan and other parts of Asia. In short order, Philadelphia became a crucible for modern medical science, public health, and eugenics reform.

In this respect, social welfare reform policy centered on the denigration of the proverbial and inconvenient "other." "Usefulness" and "improvement" were the yardstick of measuring social hierarchy and individual worth. There also were clear parallels between the segregation of African Americans and Native Americans, and the confinement of people with cognitive disability within isolated institutions. An ideology of exclusion and compulsory isolation without regard for liberty rights and basic human dignity legitimized the forced and perpetual separation of fellow citizens to facilities far removed from mainstream society. Hard as it might be to imagine, coercive institutionalization without consent was a feature of early twentieth-century reform culture at home and overseas. Proponents claimed it would be best for the individual, the family, and, more certainly, society at large.

Once thought to be progressive training facilities, institutions like Pennhurst became a nightmare, or a kind of "purgatory" for the oppressed, the epitome of what was wrong in failed public policy in the treatment of individuals with mental disabilities. Was it that these facilities had simply grown too large, and the problem of overcrowding so severe, that they proved to be unmanageable? Or, as some argued, did the very concept of perpetual institutionalization inevitably lead to abuse, medical mistreatment, and human degradation? Could it be that the very idea of Pennhurst (and similar places) contained within itself the seeds of its own ruin? Indeed, modern social scientists have found ample reason to agree with nineteenth-century reformer Samuel Gridley Howe, who helped create and develop the institutional model in America. "All great establishments in the nature of boarding schools," Howe said in 1866, "where the sexes must be separated; where there must be boarding in common, and sleeping in congregate dormitories; where there must be routine, and formality, and restraint, and repression of individuality . . . all such institutions are unnatural and undesirable, and very liable to abuse. We should have as few of them as possible, and those few should be kept as small as possible."[6]

Modern social science research has revealed how right Howe was in his observation more than a century and a half ago. Stanley Milgram found in his Yale University experiments on obedience to authority that the vast majority of subjects will "follow orders" even to the extent of harming and abusing others. Milgram demonstrated that this tendency is a nearly universal human trait: to be cruel if ordered to be cruel. Shortly thereafter, Philip Zimbardo's Stanford prison experiments on simulated prison conditions demonstrated another chilling fact about human nature: "In this study, a group of ordinary college students were divided arbitrarily into 'prisoners' and 'guards.' Hidden cameras captured what happened: the 'guards' became more sadistic, devising cruel mental tortures, while the 'prisoners' either broke down or succumbed in cowed and mindless obedience. I have to end this two-week study after only six days because it had become too real, too volatile."[7]

Similar conclusions were drawn by several psychologists who examined and extensively interviewed German war criminals during the Nuremberg Trials.[8] One should not underestimate the force of "compliance" in the therapeutic culture engendered by perpetual institutionalization. The Stanford experiment showed the inevitability of nasty and dehumanizing conditions in situations just like the ones created within large custodial institutions. They became a mirror held up to the human soul that few of us are prepared to gaze at. Also noteworthy, almost from the beginning Pennhurst and similar facilities became laboratories for medical research and human subject experimentation (see chapter 3).

With respect to perpetual institutionalization, broadcast reports by Bill Baldini at Pennhurst, Geraldo Rivera at Willowbrook, and numerous other journalist exposés created enormous unease within their viewing audiences. It wasn't just the size of these massive institutions, nor merely that the staff was bad and administrators incompetent. And it wasn't the institutions' geographic location, their architecture, or the way funds were managed. Degradation occurs when we take liberty away from a group of vulnerable people, thus branding them as "other" or "not like us." When other people are then put in a position of great power over the details of their everyday lives, and "compliance" becomes the be-all and end-all of human existence, command and control triumph in almost inevitably brutal and inhumane forms. *Order* rises to primacy at the expense of teaching, simple affection, quality of life, and human dignity. The tendency to commit atrocity is a story as old as human history, and as recent as incidents like Auschwitz and Abu Ghraib. Pennhurst, one visitor observed, "was Dachau without the ovens."

In a concrete way, the tale of Pennhurst (and similar institutions) and what it represents as one of the great transformations of American society and public values is represented in figure 1.1. For Americans with intellectual and developmental disabilities, deinstitutionalization began in about 1969. But the early wave was accomplished primarily by

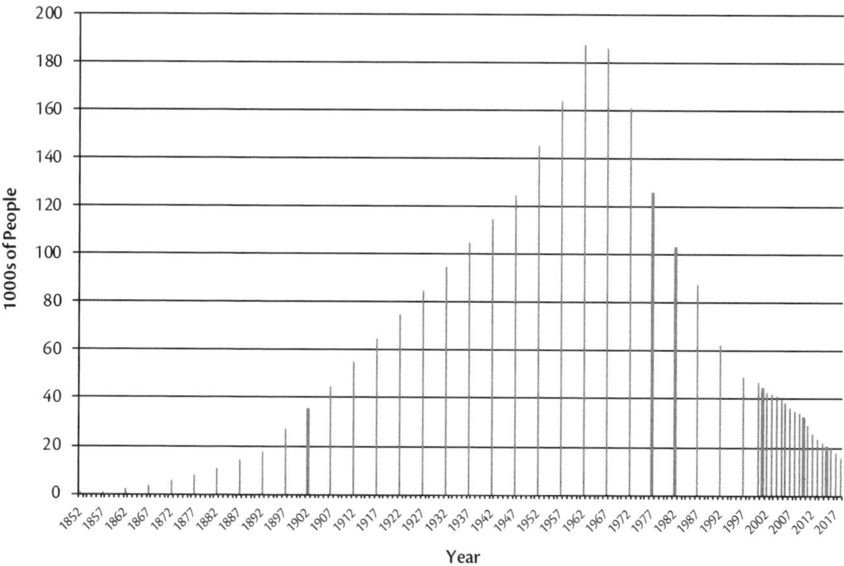


FIGURE 1.1 The number of Americans with intellectual and developmental disabilities living in public institutions, 1852–2018.

relocating people who should never have been there in the first place. This included people like Bernard Carabello at Willowbrook and thousands upon thousands of people with physical and sensory disabilities or mental illnesses who had been misplaced. The "real" movement of people with "real" intellectual disability took hold with the 1977 Pennhurst Decision. In this sense Pennhurst was the epicenter of an emerging disability rights campaign that continues to this day.

Far removed from public view, these massive custodial facilities took on an ambiance and alternative reality of their own. An industrial training school complete with an infirmary, a functioning dairy farm, a carpentry shop, an athletic and sports program, seasonal pageants, an orchestra and band, and, at least at first glance, a humane and well-ordered routine, Pennhurst seemed to offer a world of possibilities and hope for families overwhelmed by the needs of their children. But beneath this bucolic surface lurked another world of overcrowding, neglect, exploitation, and degradation. Once diminished, residents became willing targets for exploitation through medical experimentation, unknowing agents in the cause of fighting diseases like influenza, tuberculosis, and polio. Abuse and injury were routine. One of the burning questions is what happened that made things go so wrong in what many regard as a century of human progress and advanced civilization?

Outside the disability rights community, and the community of scholars interested in disability studies, there is little knowledge of the history of institutions like Pennhurst. This despite the fact institutionalization was a global phenomenon that included nearly three hundred American facilities and more than a half-million people over time.

Our intention in this volume is to tell the story of Pennhurst State School and Hospital and its place in the broader patterns of Pennsylvania and United States history. Charting the history of a single institution and its impact on social attitudes and public policy reveals a complex but largely neglected dimension of our national narrative. In fact, the Pennhurst narrative broadens into a context that reaches across the Atlantic and Pacific Oceans to create a yet-to-be-written transnational perspective on disability rights and public policy.

This narrative includes two contradictory trends—institutionalization and deinstitutionalization—and embodies one of the great, if unrecognized, freedom struggles of the twentieth century. But it also reminds us that this is a human drama filled with moments of tragedy and triumph. This story supports Arnold Toynbee's observation from more than a century ago: "History is something that happens to [other] people."[9]

This book project is the outgrowth of research and advocacy efforts that began when the Public Interest Law Center joined the Pennhurst Memorial and Preservation Alliance to dedicate the 2010 historical marker. Many of the individuals who have contributed to this volume have their own long history of involvement with Pennhurst and the disability rights movement in America. Readers may be surprised at just how complex, and how socially and politically relevant, the story of Pennhurst and other institutions is to our understanding of American history. In that respect, we hope Pennhurst invites all of us to aspire to a more complete and informed appreciation of the human dimensions of history, and the meaning of freedom, citizenship, and human rights in a democratic society.

Folklorist Charles Joyner advised that one should "ask big questions of little places." It is in this spirit that we see Pennhurst as freighted with historical and human significance. There is more to Pennhurst than Pennhurst; more than the story of one institution that operated over eight decades, and the aggregate statistics of buildings and grounds, annual budgets, and residents served. Rather than dwelling on the periphery of historical significance, the Pennhurst narrative in all of its complexity challenges us to rethink common assumptions about history, about the nature and meaning of historical progress, and about unexplored and often neglected subjects in our past. In a particular sense, as a lived experience the story of Pennhurst (and other institutions) haunts American history. How ironic that Pennhurst's crumbling buildings now host an annual Halloween Asylum venue that commercializes and takes advantage of this tortured history.

Like the historical marker ceremony, this book is an act of remembrance. The narrative includes personal testimony and recorded remembrances, and it relies on primary and secondary research in the field of disability studies. Online materials have been indispensable, and the range of source materials now accessible via the world wide web is remarkable. Wherever relevant, there has been ample use of accessible primary sources and other forms of original documentation drawn from local, regional, and national repositories. This is especially true of archives in the greater Philadelphia area. While published materials form one of the pillars of this study (along with firsthand sources and archival holdings), endnote citations have sometimes been kept to a minimum to improve the narrative flow.

We have adopted a fairly straightforward organizational structure for an eclectic and complementary set of essays. We have intentionally included both scholarly essays and more personal vignettes that emphasize how individuals and families became immersed in the historic struggles to resolve the glaring indignities that accompanied long-term incarceration. Without diminishing the scholarly value of this work, we have made the intentional decision to include the more personal voice of individuals involved in Pennhurst and disability rights and services.

What should be apparent in the larger context of disability rights is that the *personal* frequently became the *political*, and private relationships and experiences prompted both advocates and self-advocates to take a more public stand. Visiting a family member in a state institution could be an emotional, even cathartic experience. As rumors of abuse crept from the shadows, these experiences shaped efforts to dismantle the architecture of perpetual incarceration and wonton neglect.

Readers will recognize a shifting sense of tone and content that reflects the often deep personal engagement of many of the contributors to this volume. We intentionally have retained the degrees of scholarly detachment and deep personal conviction out of a respect for the human complexity that is at the heart of the Pennhurst and disability rights narratives. What results is a series of contrasting "voices" and perspectives—some personalized and some more detached—as the narrative moves from chapter to chapter.

We have divided the chapters and their contents into three broad subject areas, each with its own brief introduction. Part 1 deals with the origin and history of Pennhurst as a state institution for individuals with intellectual and developmental disabilities. Part 2 shifts the narrative to focus on Pennhurst and a growing public awareness of the shortcomings of institutionalization. These chapters discuss legal struggles and advocacy efforts by attorneys, researchers, and the families themselves. The Pennhurst Longitudinal Study tracked deinstitutionalization to assess whether residents were better off in community-based living and employment arrangements. Self-advocacy looms as a formidable force as former residents summoned the courage to speak out, organize, and address their experiences through public witness. Finally, part 3 casts an eye to current and future developments on the Pennhurst campus. They include site preservation, "urban exploration" (a new recreational activity discussed in chapter 9), and the controversial Pennhurst Asylum phenomenon, the haunted house venue that draws tens of thousands of spectators to a macabre spectacle each autumn.

Most importantly, the initiative to create a museum and interpretive center dedicated to telling the Pennhurst and disability rights saga brings the reader full circle to present-day developments.

A word or two about the problem of language and nomenclature is in order. The tendency to overgeneralize or stereotype has the effect of demeaning an individual. It may also perpetuate social stigma. "Disability" is a very broad and inclusive word that has come to refer to a vast variety of physical and mental conditions and clinical diagnoses, and it carries a very heavy political weight. "Neurodiversity" is the latest example of this tendency to mix scientific and social categories to more accurately conform to changing sensibilities and understandings of the diversity of the human condition. Sometimes the labeling is politically charged, and sometimes it reflects a bias in the search for a more complete assessment of individual traits and tendencies.

The current diagnostic preference to see autism and mental illness (depression, bipolar disorder, schizophrenia, etc.) as developmental spectrum disorders is another case in point. There is an old adage that goes "When you have met one person with a 'disability' . . . you have met one person with a disability."[10] Some activists have objected to use of the word "disability" to describe degrees of "able-ness." Inclusion—the "Inclusion Revolution"—self-determination, and person-centered are all popular phrases today.[11]

Though we cannot resolve these debates in the present study, it is important to recognize that language has always been controversial in the construction of any social identity. What are reported as clinical diagnoses often reflect the personal biases of the medical professionals who reached a kind of consensus on terminology, sometimes to suit their own agendas and professional standing. This is certainly true in the case of eugenics and the forces that gave rise to institutionalization. Over time, words like "feebleminded" and "degenerate"—or for that matter "imbeciles," "idiots," and "morons"—fell out of favor and were replaced by the phrase "mentally retarded," which in turn has been replaced by "having intellectual and developmental disabilities." Today, the word "difability" is gaining in popularity in some circles. The commonplace practice of referring to human beings as "socially inadequate," "defective," or "misfits" has fallen out of favor in polite discourse.

Words have power, and language signifies deeper social attitudes. The work at hand has as its focus the experiences of individuals with intellectual and developmental disabilities. Some readers may be more familiar with the older and now discarded phrase "mental retardation." Though grounded in the literature of disability culture studies, these essays do not center on the experiences of individuals who are blind, deaf, or who suffer from addiction, psychosis, and mental illness. We trust that readers will see the similarities and the important distinctions to be drawn.

This history of Pennhurst State School and Hospital begins with the themes of isolation and exclusion, the intentional creation of a world apart. (That movement had a more sinister component as well.) It concludes with a countermovement away from institutionalization and toward greater inclusion in the mainstream. The return of individuals to Community Living Arrangements (CLAs) is one of the great unheralded transformations in modern life, and it has global implications. But it is a revolution that is not without its own social, economic, and cultural problems and challenges, and it has profound public policy implications. Such is the arc of disability history in contemporary America.

This is a cautionary tale still filled with enormous uncertainty, and it has a relevance to present-day policy debates about "person-centered" support services. It is also about individual worth, citizens' rights, and the "place" of people with disabilities in contemporary society. This is a narrative that is not yet ended, and as such it brings the past and the present into relationship through the prism of one place and its people, with the hope of creating a better future. Tragedy and triumph, memory and hope—these are the boundaries of history as lived experience, and they frame this complex story in a context of local, national, and international significance.

## Notes

1. *Tragedy and Triumph: Telling the Pennhurst Story, A Marker Dedication* (Philadelphia: Pennsylvania Humanities Council, 2010), 59.

2. Ibid.

3. *Map of State and Semi-State Institutions of Pennsylvania* (Philadelphia: Public Charities Association of Pennsylvania, ca. 1923). Original on deposit at Pennsylvania State Archives; copy in author's possession.

4. Dennis B. Downey, "'Detect Early; Protect Always': Philadelphia Physcians and the Gospel of Eugenics," *Pennsylvania Legacies* 17 (Fall 2017): 12–19.

5. Halderman v. Pennhurst State School and Hospital, 446 F. Supp. 1295.

6. Samuel G. Howe in 1866 ceremonies on laying the cornerstone of the New York State Institution for the Blind at Batavia, Genessee County, New York. Quoted in G. Garrell, *The Story of Blindness* (Cambridge: Harvard University Press, 2009).

7. C. Haney, C. Banks, and P. Zambardo, "Interpersonal Dynamics in a Simulated Prison," *International Journal of Criminology and Penology* 1, no. 1 (1973): 69–97.

8. Joel E. Dimsdale, *Anatomy of Malice: The Enigma of Nazi War Criminals* (New Haven: Yale University Press, 2016), 155–97.

9. Quoted in C. Vann Woodward, *Origins of the New South, 1877–1913*, 1951 (Baton Rouge: Louisiana State University Press, rev. ed. 1981), frontispiece, n.p.

10. Steve Silberman, *NeuroTribes: The Legacy of Autism and the Future of Neurodiversity* (New York: Penguin Random House, 2015); John Donvan and Caren Zucker, *In a Different Key: The Story of Autism* (New York: Crown, 2016), 191–327; Ron Powers, *No One Cares About Crazy People* (New York: Hachette Books, 2017), 21–38.

11. On the limitations of "mentally retarded" as a social and diagnostic typology, see Rick Hodges, "The Rise and Fall of the 'Mentally Retarded': How a Term That Replaced Bad Words Became One—and How to Stop It from Happening Again," *Medium*, July 10, 2015, https://medium.com/s/story/the-rise-and-fall-of-mentally-retarded-e3b9eea23018.

PART 1

# Pennhurst in Time and Place

Part 1 explains the origins and history of Pennhurst in the context of the institutionalization of people with intellectual and developmental disabilities. These institutions were large-scale facilities that were state government operated or funded. They reflected the social attitudes and political agenda of their creators. In the United States, they grew until there were nearly three hundred institutions or so-called training schools, and over the decades they housed more than a half-million citizens who were deprived of their liberty and constitutional rights.

Institutionalization became a source of national shame due to inhumane overcrowding, underfunding, and chronic understaffing. These shortcomings led to wanton abuse and neglect on a massive national scale. "A snake pit," Senator Robert Kennedy said after visiting several New York institutions in the mid-1960s. With a deliberate focus on Pennhurst, part 1 shows how from the very beginning perpetual incarceration was an inherently flawed social policy and secretive in nature. Control, coercion, and compliance were the order of the day. Hidden from the mainstream, state institutions were a deliberate outcome of political willfulness, and they bore more than incidental similarity to internment and concentration camps, and other forms of legalized segregation. Justice Thurgood Marshall saw the similarities and in 1985 declared that institutions for citizens with mental disabilities exceeded the worst features of Jim Crow racial segregation.

CHAPTER 1

# The Idea of Pennhurst

## *Eugenics and the Abandonment of Hope*

DENNIS B. DOWNEY

> The first duty of medicine is not to cure disease, but to prevent it.
>
> —MAJOR LEONARD DARWIN, 1926[1]

Charles Harrison Frazier, MD (1870–1936), was a pillar of the Philadelphia establishment, one of its proverbial "best men" and an icon in the field of modern medical science. Although few individuals today outside the medical profession would know his name, Frazier had a tremendous influence on surgical practices and medical education. By the early twentieth century, he had achieved a reputation as a surgical pioneer, educator, and dean of the prestigious University of Pennsylvania School of Medicine. Frazier was a leading figure in that remarkable generation of American physicians who helped to usher in an era of modern medical research and public health policy. He also was an ardent social reformer in the public charities movement, a tireless advocate of public health and hygiene as the wellspring of individual fitness and social progress. A man of science with seemingly boundless energy and interests, Frazier authored scores of medical articles, including a brief but provocative 1908 pamphlet entitled *The Menace of the Feebleminded in Pennsylvania.*[2]

What most alarmed Frazier and his colleagues in the Public Charities Association of Pennsylvania and across the United States was the rising tide of hereditary feeblemindedness (commonly called "idiots," "morons," and "imbeciles"), what today would be termed intellectual disability, and its perilous social consequences.[3] In league with other physicians, scientists, and university researchers, they forged a new consensus, a new descriptive terminology that redefined the purpose of institutionalization as a permanent preventative measure aimed at protecting society from those who threatened biological and social progress. "Detect early / Protect always" became the guiding principle of mass institutionalization for life. In short order a model of coercive care displaced an older paradigm of compassionate treatment, training, and uplift. At the cutting edge of a national and international movement, their medical ethics and social conservatism sanctioned a series of reforms that shaped disability policy for generations to come. Years before Madison Grant, Lothrop Stoddard, and J. H. Kellogg warned of the urgency of racial hygiene, Philadelphia scientists and policy makers preached a gospel of eugenics as the surest means of biological improvement and race survival.[4]

According to a 1910 U.S. Bureau of the Census report, feebleminded referred to "all degrees of mental defect due to arrested or imperfect mental development as a result of which the person so afflicted is incapable of competing on equal terms with his normal fellows, or managing himself or his affairs with ordinary prudence." In other words, someone who had a permanent cognitive deficiency that limited their mental age to between two and twelve years of age. Self-sufficiency, independence, and "improvement" were said to be out of the question. That year, more than sixty institutions in thirty-one states provided permanent care for feebleminded and epileptic citizens, and the numbers were growing.[5]

According to the 1890 federal census, Pennsylvania had the largest number of feebleminded citizens in the United States (8,753).[6] Less than two decades later, Frazier and his peers used the federal census to assert that number had increased to eighteen thousand "mental defectives," nearly half of whom were wayward young women of childbearing age. Their cognitive impairment, it was alleged, was accompanied by a heightened degree of sexual promiscuity, criminality, and moral degradation. Perhaps most unsettling, the alleged increase in feeblemindedness, epilepsy, and other mental defects was perceived to be a national and international crisis that showed no indication of abatement or decline.

No lone wolf or isolated voice, Charles Frazier and other Philadelphia physicians promoted an ideology of care in turn-of-the century Philadelphia that brought physicians, social workers, psychologists, public hygiene proponents, and politicians into a municipal alliance to combat impediments to social progress. Many of these medical professionals (like Frazier) were educated at the University of Pennsylvania Medical College or Jefferson Medical College, and they practiced in the city. (Still others, like H. H. Goddard and E. G. Conklin, were educated at the finest graduate schools in America.) As medical pioneers and social engineers (in the Progressive reform sense), Philadelphia physicians worked with their political allies at the local and state level to enact legislation aimed at eliminating the causes and debilitating effects of crime, pauperism, sexual promiscuity, and other vices.

"I believe," Charles Frazier wrote at the dawn of the American Century, "that the most important problem we have before us is that of the prevention of mental defect." (It was more important than infant mortality, sanitation, contagious disease, impure milk and water, and a slew of other concerns.) The Public Charities Association, the American Philosophical Society, and the municipal Department of Public Health—Philadelphia's elite establishment in general—were willing institutional collaborators in eliminating the root cause of hereditary "defect," which they likened to the public enemy number one in public health.

To support his woeful medical jeremiad, Frazier cited a series of ongoing investigations conducted by Philadelphia's Board of Public Health and Charities, and the research of professed experts in the field like Martin Barr, MD, and H. H. Goddard, PhD. The municipal investigations resulted in a half-dozen reports (1910–13) under the guidance of Joseph S. Neff, MD, Philadelphia's director of the board of health. His conclusions were remarkably similar to the findings of a British Royal Commission report also released in 1908—incidentally the year Pennhurst opened. Like other leaders in the Philadelphia medical community, Charles Frazier accepted the prevailing belief that feeblemindedness was overwhelmingly an inherited and incurable *defect* (his word) that had ruinous personal and social consequences in what Charles Darwin had termed the great "struggle for existence." Purportedly empirical evidence—science and medical research—supported a widely held belief that 75 percent of the afflicted had inherited the condition from one or both parents, and all were capable of passing it on to their children. Social theorist Charles Davenport put it more crudely when he advised that the time had come to "dry up the streams . . . of defective and degenerate protoplasm"—in short, bad blood.[7]

"Defectives," "deviants," and "degenerates" were common terms within medical circles and in the popular press. Although such terminology is inflammatory today, the terms appeared regularly in public discourse, and in public health publications and enabling legislation. In Philadelphia and elsewhere, there existed a broad consensus that hereditary mental and moral defect—what Isaac Newton Kerlin, MD, termed mental and moral "imbecility"—went hand in hand: "It [defect] is definitely inherited, according to the best scientific thought of our day," Frazier wrote. "Idiocy is not a disease," Martin Barr, a Penn-trained physician and superintendent of the Pennsylvania Training School at Elwyn, insisted, "it is a defect" that is passed on from generation to generation.[8] Like his mentor Kerlin, another Penn graduate, Martin Barr based his conclusion on decades of personal observation and categorization of Elwyn residents. He, like Kerlin, treated the children in his charge as laboratory specimens used to construct the working hypothesis of hereditary feeblemindedness. "True Feeble-mindedness is not curable . . . and it is strongly inheritable," echoed E. R. Johnstone, an ally and superintendent of the Training School in Vineland, New Jersey.[9]

Philadelphia Director of Public Health Dr. Joseph S. Neff, a Penn and Jefferson Medical College graduate who achieved national prominence in public health circles, agreed. Neff supervised public health investigations, and he authored a series of pamphlets, one of which dealt specifically with the "threat" of young women unable to control their sexual impulses. His conclusions could be sweeping and over-generalized, but they conformed to standard views about unchecked procreation. Writing in 1910, Neff and his investigators asserted that "feeble-minded women produce many children. . . . Most of the children of feeble-minded women are either illegitimate or feeble-minded or both."[10] These offspring posed an intolerable economic burden, and a sure "social evil" if their promiscuity was left uncheck.

Speaking to University of Pennsylvania faculty in 1917 (ten years before the United States Supreme Court ruled "three generations of imbeciles is enough"), Charles Frazier asserted that the number of the feebleminded women of childbearing age in Philadelphia had nearly doubled in the previous decade to over 3,200. "The abnormal fecundity of the feeble-minded and mental defective," he said, "has been proven over and over again in statistical studies in every country here and abroad." Prisons were overpopulated, the courts overburdened, and "the defectives are almost inevitably recidivists and therefore doubly expensive to the taxpayers." "Owing to the fecundity of feeble-minded women," wrote a sympathetic Frazier, "the proportion will increase unless vigorous preventive measures be adopted and enforced."[11] As if to bring home the point, Martin Barr scolded that for this so-called "grotesque travesty of humanity," society cannot replace what nature never placed at the outset.[12]

As early as 1902, a year before a new state facility in Chester County received legislative approval, Barr lamented that the crusade for *usefulness* had failed and a new professional consensus had taken hold: "We have trained," he said of the physicians who worked directly with the feebleminded, "[but] for—what? There is yet, I believe, a consensus that abandons the *hope* long cherished of a return of the imbecile to the world."[13] What is to be done with the feeble-minded and epileptic?" Charles Frazier asked. "How shall we deal with them?" How might society protect itself from this scourge, or, to use Frazier's term, "increasing numbers of helpless defectives" who posed a "menace" by their very existence?

This loss of hope among medical experts was critical in the triumph of a new model of permanent custodial care that opened the door to massive state-owned facilities and the perpetual segregation and confinement of those diagnosed as unworthy of living in the community.

At the turn of the twentieth century, medical doctors in Philadelphia and around the country, and overseas, cast children and adults with intellectual disabilities as human misfits and miscreants. Princeton biologist and future American Philosophical Society president Edwin Grant Conklin called them "mistakes"—and viewed them as a biological and social contaminant to the gene pool and to future human progress. At the dawn of the Progressive Era—an era of reform and regulation—science, public health, and government policy coalesced around new public policy and standards of ethical treatment aimed at eliminating disability. Some public intellectuals and policymakers went further, with an often unspoken desire to eliminate people with disabilities themselves. Their solutions were naïve and misguided, and frequently more sinister.

## Eugenics and Public Health

Pennhurst must be understood as a creature of modernity, the direct result of modern medical science and public health policy. Similarly, as the foregoing section illustrates, Pennhurst and the nearly three hundred state institutions for the treatment of the feebleminded and epileptics flourished in the age of eugenic thought. However, neither Pennhurst nor any other public facility would have existed without the *political will* to create and sustain massive residential complexes for the perpetual "incarceration" of its inmates. This convergence of modern science, eugenics, and public health reform—"illiberal" reform as one scholar put it—was one of the most striking developments in public policy in the so-called Progressive Era (1890–1915).[14]

A full descriptive history of the rise and decline of eugenic thought is beyond the scope of this chapter, and there is a well-established literature on eugenics' impact on scientific and social thought.[15] Immigration policy, race theory, and social attitudes toward those judged to be unfit reflected eugenic thinking. A diverse group of social and corporate elites championed eugenics and its application to social and economic conditions, including Alexander Graham Bell, Theodore

Roosevelt, Woodrow Wilson, Havelock Ellis, Margaret Sanger, J. H. Kellogg, Edward and Mary Harriman, members of the Rockefeller family, novelist Edgar Rice Burroughs, race theorists Madison Grant and Lothrop Stoddard, and the elder Oliver Wendell Holmes and his namesake. This group included many of America's leading medical professionals, academics, and public intellectuals.

The Eugenics Records Office (ERO) at Cold Spring Harbor, New York, and its steady stream of pamphlets, reports, and a journal entitled *Eugenics News*, served as a national clearinghouse. Under the leadership of Charles Davenport and Harry Laughlin, the ERO advocated for legislative solutions and sponsored research on the social problems associated with hereditary defect. An estimated two hundred American colleges offered courses on eugenics-related topics; eugenic theory transformed research and instruction in biology, history, economics, psychology, and other disciplines. Prestigious universities like Johns Hopkins, Princeton, Chicago, Stanford, and the University of Pennsylvania had renowned faculty who published regularly on eugenics themes. Suffice it to say, eugenics resonated across a broad ideological spectrum, and it cast a long shadow over twentieth-century American and European social policy.[16]

A cottage industry of sorts grew up in both Europe and the United States as eugenic ideas became acceptable in highbrow and popular culture. Eugenic thinking permeated Sabbath sermons and holiday festivals. Professional organizations, book clubs, publishing houses, international conferences and colloquia, and research institutes provided an outlet for like-minded specialists to advance notions of heredity and human development. The American Breeders' Association, Eugenics Society, and J. Harvey Kellogg's Battle Creek Sanitarium and its program for "biologic living" and "race betterment" attracted wide public notice. Summertime "Better Baby" and "Fitter Family" contests—the forerunners of beauty pageants—became the rage at county and state fairs. In many states medical exams became a precondition for securing a marriage license.

A short-lived American Eugenics Party promoted a decidedly conservative legislative agenda at the state and national level. International Eugenics Conferences held periodically between 1912 and 1936 attracted a veritable who's who of prominent scientists, social theorists, medical professionals, and racial hygiene purists from America and across Europe. Major Leonard Darwin, Charles's son and a leader of the British Eugenics Society, occupied a prestigious position. At meetings held in London, New York, and Berlin, American eugenicists collaborated with German racial hygienists and kept up a regular correspondence on progress in the field. In 1936, the ERO's Harry Laughlin received an honorary degree from Heidelberg University for his advocacy work, most notably in the area of state sterilization legislations.

Euphemistically called the "science of better breeding," eugenics rose to prominence in the decades following the 1859 appearance of Charles Darwin's revolutionary book *On the Origin of Species*. Darwin's cousin Francis Galton, the author of the widely read *Hereditary Genius* (1869), is generally credited as the "father of eugenics," and for giving heredity a more explicit and formidable role in human evolution. Like Charles Darwin and his son Leonard, Galton was fascinated by variation within a species, and especially the ability of the human species to pass on desirable and undesirable traits.

In the halcyon days of the new century, eugenic thought permeated American public discourse and cut a wide swath through highbrow and popular culture. From the pulpit to the judicial bench, and in many a state legislature, eugenic thought shaped social, political, and even judicial attitudes toward those said to be of inferior or defective stock. In a moment of poetic inspiration, Virginia public health physician John H. Bell wrote in 1930 (three years after the Supreme Court upheld the constitutionality of sterilization in *Buck v. Bell*): "The buds unfit to mature, fall; / And the weaklings of the flock must perish."[17]

Francis Galton and his disciples were as indebted to Thomas Malthus and his theory of overpopulation as they were to a scientific basis for human biological degradation. Eugenicists had a penchant for statistics, and for categorizing and classifying the degrees of mental "defect," and they created their own language and terminology to describe the nature and degree of human decay.[18] With an eye to future generations, supporters of Galton's belief in heredity popularized a more proactive intervention through engineering human reproduction to weed out undesirable traits that jeopardized social and biological progress. As Galton himself explained in 1908, the year Pennhurst opened: "Its [eugenics'] first object is to check the birth-rate of the Unfit, instead of allowing them to come into being, though doomed in large numbers to perish prematurely."[19] Weeks later, Galton wrote a widely circulated editorial in the *London Times* that asserted there was now ample evidence that "the bulk of the community was deteriorating."[20]

Eugenicists on both sides of the Atlantic Ocean stressed that *intelligence* and *ability* had an acquired component that was passed down through generations. If genius is inheritable, was not its opposite? It was a simple proposition that reinforced conservative social views. Diminished mental ability thwarted nature's design and therefore jeopardized order. Mental and moral "defect" were incapable of *improvement* and left unchecked would interfere with both biological and social progress.

As Leonard Darwin observed, and as fellow eugenicists campaigned, prevention and proactive solutions were essential. Human reproduction, and its encouragement among the "fit" and its denial among the "unfit," was the key. In the rough and tumble of a struggle for existence, it was not too far of a stretch to equate fit and unfit with levels of mental and moral acumen. As his biographer noted, Galton came to believe that "physical features reflected specific behavioral or racial traits" that led to immorality, sexual excessiveness, crime, and pauperism, to name just a few.[21]

Much like other species, selective human breeding was an essential element of "eugenic science." Sexual and social "mixing" with those groups judged to be inferior on the mental, moral, and behavioral spectrum became taboo (and sometimes illegal). Parallels to racial attitudes are striking. In a real sense, such theory revolved around a sense of place and status, and an ominous devotion to theories of biological purity. Heredity became the basis for understanding, categorizing, and ameliorating the conditions that impeded both biological purity and social progress. It also served as the inspiration to a vogue of genealogical or family studies aimed at demonstrating how physical, mental, and social deviancy reappeared generation after generation.[22]

Ironically, the apostles of eugenics looked to the past (family lineage) to safeguard the future from biological or genetic contaminates.

"To purify the breeding stock of the race at all costs is the slogan of eugenics," declared Harry Laughlin.[23] "We are assuming," he wrote in a far-ranging report, "for this particular study that heredity as an important factor in the production of defectives and in the causation of anti-social conduct is a fact and is generally accepted by the American people."[24] Not only did such thinking reinforce a sense of social hierarchy based on inheritance and intelligence, it served to define the "place" of individuals with intellectual and developmental disabilities—indeed people with any disability—as social outsiders unfit for normal human associations. Martin Barr was forthright in favoring the "free use of the pruning knife" to arrest unwelcome "perversions" (both sexual and behavioral). His one-time colleague at Elwyn (and fellow-Kerlin disciple) A. W. Wilmarth, MD, wrote of the "sins of ancestry . . . unbridled by the control of a moral sense." Another Philadelphia physician and author, acclaimed Jefferson Medical College surgeon J. Ewing Mears was even more aggressive in supporting sterilization as a therapeutic means of "stopping the flow of degeneracy" as a condition for what he called "race betterment."[25] Each lecturer championed the winnowing out or elimination of a dissolute population of defective human beings whose very existence posed an obstacle to future progress.

Over two decades, more than twenty states adopted statutes that empowered state officials, acting on the advice of physician boards, to curtail the ability of the feebleminded to reproduce. In Europe, Denmark, Norway, Finland, Sweden, and England approved compulsory sterilization statutes. Buoyed by eugenics, German racial theorists embraced a more radical and exterminationist ideology for what they argued was "life unfit for life." Thc infamous T4 Program that isolated and subsequently euthanized children and adults with disabilities was a pretext for the Holocaust. Each demonstrated the willingness of physicians, nurses, and other medical professionals to cross ethical boundaries in the service of medical science and public policy. This new sensibility represented the triumph of political will over moral courage in the Holocaust era.[26]

More reserved in their approach to eliminating individuals with mental disabilities, American and Pennsylvania medical and political leaders embraced a three-part solution to answer Charles Frazier's question, "What is to be done?": not extermination but elimination through sterilization, segregation through institutionalization, and regulating the right to marry. The objective was to eliminate the condition by attacking the root of the problem: the ability to reproduce. Thus would be created not just a world without disability but a world without the disabled themselves. The fallacious perspective put science and new surgical techniques in the service of an illusory social progress and biological improvement.

It is noteworthy that the first documented sterilizations of so-called feebleminded individuals occurred in Pennsylvania. Prior to 1900, at least 279 involuntary sterilization procedures were performed at the Pennsylvania Training School at Elwyn, and perhaps more were done at facilities in western Pennsylvania.[27] Isaac Kerlin saw the procedure ("oophorectomy" and "orchotomia") as necessary "for the relief and cure of radical depravity."[28] He championed the experimental surgery in public addresses and in print, and by his own admission he was performing the procedure years earlier. Kerlin's protégé Martin Barr praised "the free use of the pruning knife. . . . It is a war of extermination." Their neighbor J. E. Mears, MD, thought sterilization "remedial and curative," and a tool in the struggle for "race betterment."

Such medical intervention was performed in the shadows without public fanfare, and none were performed with informed consent or legal authorization. His "pets," as Kerlin called the children approaching puberty, were his wards, and sterilization served a greater public good. Many thought so-called asexualization, which included tubal ligation and castration, had a calming effect and curbed antisocial behaviors in criminals, sexual deviants, and the feebleminded. Many physicians thought it also limited masturbation and other aggressive impulses. Compulsory sterilization would be best for everyone.

Though Indiana is credited with being the first among two dozen states to enact involuntary sterilization laws for people with intellectual disabilities (1907), almost two decades earlier the first of a half-dozen sexual sterilization bills was introduced into the Pennsylvania General

Assembly. Though stymied in each attempt, proponents continued their efforts to secure passage over twenty years. In each instance the medical community, and public health officials in Philadelphia, rallied to the cause. (In all, more than sixty thousand American citizens underwent involuntary sterilizations between 1907 and 1980; California and North Carolina led the way.)

In 1905 the Pennsylvania General Assembly passed a bill entitled "An Act For the Prevention of Idiocy." True to the eugenic consensus, its first line read: "Whereas, Heredity plays a most important part in the transmission of idiocy and imbecility." Though approved by the legislature, the proposed statute was vetoed by Governor Samuel Pennypacker. His message to the legislature was blunt: "Scientists, like all other men whose experiences have been limited to one pursuit, and whose minds have been developed in a particular direction, sometimes need to be restrained. . . . To permit such an operation would be to inflict cruelty upon a helpless class in the community, which the State has undertaken to protect." With a swipe at Martin Barr, who had advocated for the legislation in the pages of *Heredity* magazine, Pennypacker found it unconscionable for the government to perpetrate such practices on human subjects, especially without their informed consent (which was neither required nor possible). The governor showed no such qualms about institutionalizing the feebleminded when he signed the Pennhurst bill in the previous session.[29]

Following five other failed attempts, an involuntary sterilization bill sponsored by Philadelphia State Senator G. Stanley Woodward, MD, did pass the state assembly in 1921. Governor William Sproul followed Pennypacker's example and vetoed the legislation, though it had the support of state and national public health officials and the endorsement of the Eugenics Research Lab at Cold Spring Harbor. Though an early leader in the campaign, Pennsylvania never enacted a state-sanctioned sterilization law.

With the public support for sterilization waning, a complementary strategy for preventing feeblemindedness in Pennsylvania gained momentum in the public health community. As early as 1912, Director Joseph Neff outlined twelve legislative initiatives in his annual report to the Philadelphia Department of Public Health and Charities. Even as he lamented the defeat of a 1911 bill "to prevent the procreation of idiots, imbeciles, and feeble-minded persons by the process of sterilization," Neff voiced enthusiasm for a related initiative. Public health officials would support "an Act to prevent the marriage of the unfit, which is necessary to prevent the deterioration of future generations." A physician himself, Neff recommended a vigorous effort to educate the public and state legislators on "the importance of such an Act from an economic standpoint before there would be likelihood of passage."[30] The so-called "antimixing" statute, which resembled antimiscegenation statutes in the era, effectively criminalized sexual relations with or between one or more people determined to be mentally defective. Try as they did on several occasions, physician-advocates and their political allies were unsuccessful in securing passage of a ban on sexual union as a means to prevent procreation.

The third and perhaps most acceptable strategy to control a growing population of feebleminded children and adults involved a redefinition of a long-standing practice of institutionalization. In state after state—nearly three hundred facilities in total—institutions were constructed and maintained well off the beaten path and far removed from public view. They were part of what David Rothman termed the century-long "discovery of the asylum." Another student of the trend termed residents "inconvenient people."[31] By 1923, Pennsylvania was providing direct care and full financial support to nearly sixty state-operated custodial facilities, and subsidies to aid a handful of private institutions like the Training School at Elwyn.

Five of these state institutions were dedicated to individuals judged to be "mentally defective" and feebleminded, or epileptic. The largest facilities were the Western State Institution for the Feeble-Minded (created in 1893 and opened in 1897) at Polk in rural Venango County, and the Eastern Pennsylvania State Institution for the Feeble-Minded, which was approved in 1903 and opened in 1908. Renamed the Pennhurst State School and Hospital in the 1920s, the sprawling campus sat in rural Chester County more than twenty-five miles from Center City Philadelphia. Judging by the legislative history, and according to Charles Frazier and other advocates, institutionalization was politically the most palatable solution to the perceived rising tide of feeblemindedness.[32]

The consensus had formed years before Pennhurst came into existence. Speaking to an overflow crowd attending the National Charities Conference that met during the 1893 World's Columbian Exposition in Chicago, social work advocate George H. Knight put the matter succinctly: "We must have institutions for this class, both for their sake and for the sake of the community."[33] In 1911, W. W. Hawke, MD, told a Philadelphia symposium, "All feeble minded (referring to those mentally deficient from birth or early infancy) should be placed in an institution for life. The State should provide separate institutions for this particular type of individual, and in no instance should they be confined in the several insane asylums or almshouses for the care of the dependent." Once detained, Hawke argued, "Asexualization is advisable under proper regulation."[34] A year later, preeminent eugenicist Charles Davenport insisted society must end "in one way or another these animalistic blood-lines or they will end society."[35]

Edwin G. Conklin, the Johns Hopkins–trained biologist who taught at Princeton University before ascending to the presidency of Philadelphia's American Philosophical Society, wrote in *the Journal of Heredity* (1915) of the feebleminded as human "mistakes" and society's need for "eugenical insurance against having defective children."[36] According to Conklin and his public health colleagues, custodial incarceration in state institutions like Polk and Pennhurst was the most effect way to decrease "the number of defectives born from defective parents."[37]

Built to address Philadelphia concerns and to relieve overcrowding elsewhere, the Eastern Pennsylvania State Institution for the Feebleminded and Epileptic (Pennhurst State School and Hospital) reflected the convergence of eugenics and a new model of institutionalization.[38] Gone was an older tradition of compassionate care championed by Dorothea Dix and Samuel Gridley Howe, replaced by what each loathed: sprawling and impersonal facilities geared toward a culture of compliance and rules. Experts like Charles Frazier foolishly believed such an approach would be more cost effective. Over eight decades more than 10,600 individuals were "incarcerated" within Pennhurst's walls.

Signed into law by Governor Pennypacker on May 15, 1903, Public Law No. 424 authorized commissioners to select a site far removed from any population center but like Polk "accessible by railroad facilities to the counties of Eastern Pennsylvania." Final approval of all site plans, including buildings and infrastructure, architectural design, and the cottage-style layout then in vogue was subject to the consent of the State Board of Charities. In short order charities officials approved a site on Crab Hill outside Spring City in Chester County.

Committing residents with mental disabilities to the status of social outsiders, the 1903 law carefully regulated the physical space and the *place* of inhabitants within the walls. "The buildings shall be in two groups, one for the educational or industrial department, and one for the custodial or asylum department." With an eye to future needs, the legislature included provisions for expansion as the population grew beyond an initial five hundred residents to over three thousand fifty years later. Parents could voluntarily commit their children provided they bore at least some of the expense, or (more commonly) commitment would occur through a legal process supported by a physician's recommendation. True to the prevailing institutional model, the superintendent had to be a physician with a minimum of five years of experience in the field.

Any child under the age of twenty who was "incapable of receiving instruction in the common schools of the State" was eligible to become an "inmate." Misdiagnosis was common. Adults adjudged to be feebleminded (or epileptic) "and who are of such inoffensive habits as to make them proper subjects" could be involuntarily incarcerated following the guidelines established for state mental hospitals. Puberty seems to have been the critical threshold. The criteria for committal were so elastic as to permit a large and heterogeneous population, thus helping to explain the rapid growth in the custodial population. Once committed and a ward of the state, consensual rights were lost, including the right to leave. Runaways invariably were returned.[39]

Reinforcing the sense of social isolation and compulsory quarantine, the legislature included language meant to assure that Pennhurst was self-sustaining. Residents who were able would be assigned to the workroom, to dairy and agricultural labor, and to cleaning the dormitories, offices, and washrooms. It also came to include watching over fellow residents and providing personal hygiene. Those unable to demonstrate their "usefulness" or "self-sufficiency" were consigned to the catch-all custodial department. This two-tiered population (industrial and custodial) became more fixed as the numbers increased, and especially after women were committed to Pennhurst. By the 1950s and in the face of chronic understaffing and inadequate services, working residents existing in a state of virtual peonage helped assure an annual profit of $25,000 to $50,000.[40]

Always, however, the ironclad rule of segregating the sexes had to be maintained lest the larger purpose of preventing reproduction collapse. Section 10 of the statute made this clear: "That this institution shall be entirely and specially devoted to the reception, detention, care and training of the epileptics and of the idiotic and feeble-minded persons, of either sex, and shall be so planned in the beginning and construction, as shall provide separate classification of the numerous groups embraced under the terms 'epileptics' and 'idiotic" and 'imbecile' or 'feeble-minded.'" In this regard Pennhurst was not exceptional; the designers were following the prevailing wisdom in the field. Women, when they were placed at Pennhurst, lived in separate buildings within the larger compound.

Within three years of receiving its first resident in November 1908, complaints circulated of overcrowding, inadequate funding, and neglect at Pennhurst. On the advice of Joseph Neff, state officials acted. "A proper regard for the public welfare requires that some action be taken looking to the segregation of such feeble-minded and epileptic persons." At the behest of public health officials, in 1911 Governor John Tener and the General Assembly appointed a statewide "commission on the Segregation, Care and Treatment of the Feeble-Minded and Epileptic Persons."[41]

The commission released its findings two years later, and they read like a textbook primer for applied eugenics. In recommendation after recommendation, the report echoed what Philadelphia physicians had been saying for years. This should not be surprising, since Joseph Neff (commission president), Samuel G. Dixon (director, Pennsylvania Department of Public Health), and other Philadelphia-based physicians, and their hand-picked consultants, had prominent roles in the commission work. One of the key recommendations stated:

"Segregation of the feeble-minded of the institutional type, however, will continue to remain the principal means of protection which society can provide. Sterilization may be more effective and more economical than segregation [to halt reproduction]."[42]

Like Charles H. Frazier, these commissioners remained committed to a policy of compulsory sexual sterilization of "feeble-minded women of child-bearing age," who constituted a "grave social menace." Officials drew a distinction between the care of the "teachable," a distinct minority, and the overwhelming majority of "defectives" who were classified as hereditary "idiots." Regarding women of childbearing age, the commission "is firmly convinced that sterilization, or compulsory, custodial provision of such character as to prevent further increase of mental defectives (or both) should be provided for. The time appears to have come when the state, for its own protection, is compelled to assume control over a class which is now spreading immorality and disease, and which is steadily increasing the number of defective delinquents and criminals."[43] Two dozen years before Justice Oliver Wendell Holmes Jr. declared in *Buck v. Bell* (1927) that "three generations of imbeciles is enough," Pennsylvania officials had reached a similar conclusion.[44]

With a waiting list of over five thousand eligible clients for permanent custodial placement (or confinement), the commission recommended the legislature appropriate funds for a dramatic building program. With a 1911 capacity of five hundred, Pennhurst was to be tripled in size over the next fifteen years, chiefly to accommodate feebleminded young women at or near the age of puberty. Additional dormitories and other facilities should be constructed as well. Commissioners recommended a new statute "defining insanity and feeble-mindedness as forms of mental unsoundness, and placing all indigent mental defectives under the care of the State." Clearer "methods of commitment, detention, support, parole, and discharge of all forms of mental unsoundness in Pennsylvania" were needed.[45]

As Joseph Neff wrote, custodial incarceration was in the "public interest," and it was the most politically tenable way to prevent and eliminate hereditary feeblemindedness. Segregation as a means to prevent human reproduction became the acceptable solution to what

Charles Frazier had termed an "increasingly desperate situation." Just four years after the 1913 report, and with Pennhurst poised for expansion, Frazier asserted, "Feeble-mindedness is an inherited and incurable condition. Once feeble-minded, always feeble-minded. . . . The only protection for the next generation is segregation." Prevention, not cure, was the path to social progress, and in true eugenic fashion, it required the isolation and gradual elimination of human beings whose very existence undermined the social order.

Medical doctors, scientists, and an educated elite—professional *experts* in the field—showed the way. In the bargain, basic liberty was the price to pay. This was the idea that brought Pennhurst into existence, and it shaped early twentieth-century public policy on disability and citizenship. Segregation, quarantine, or removal, call it what you will, this was the social policy disability rights advocates would struggle against for generations to come. No matter that the price was a loss of social identity, human dignity, and constitutional rights for fellow citizens. Institutionalization was now part of public policy.

Just two years before Pennhurst released its last resident to community living in 1987, Supreme Court Justice Thurgood Marshall wrote a blistering rebuke of the institutionalization of individuals with intellectual disabilities. He decried what he called "a regime of *state-mandated* segregation and degradation . . . that in its virulence and bigotry rivaled, and indeed paralleled, the worst excesses of Jim Crow [racial segregation]." Their purpose, he correctly concluded, was to "halt reproduction of the retarded and 'nearly extinguish their race.'"[46] No stranger to the freedom struggles of the civil rights era, Marshall recognized the inherent dangers in warehousing human beings without constitutional protections.

Long after a eugenics-inspired campaign had fallen out of favor, massive custodial institutions like Pennhurst continued to exist at enormous human and financial costs. Ironically, and perhaps tragically, it was public exposure of abuse and the deplorable—Justice Marshall said "grotesque"—conditions of life within Pennhurst's walls that helped launch a parallel freedom struggle that is ongoing today. In the post–World War II era, court litigation over conditions at Pennhurst transformed American constitutional law and public policy. Family and organizational advocacy, and the force of investigative reporting, propelled Pennhurst and similar institutions to center stage in a national and then global disability civil rights movement that marked a reversal, if not a complete repudiation, of the corrosive disability policies enacted at the dawn of the American Century.

## Notes

1. Leonard Darwin, *The Need for Eugenic Reform* (New York: D. Appleton, 1926), 196.

2. Charles H. Frazier, *The Menace of the Feeble-Minded in Pennsylvania*, Publication 7 (Philadelphia: Public Charities Association, 1908); "Dr. Frazier Recommends Segregation of Feeble-Minded," *Pennsylvania Gazette* 15, no. 7 (February 1917): 164–67.

3. "Feebleminded" was a catch-all diagnostic phrase that referred to a hierarchy or degree of mental deficiency, literally from low- to high-grade function. Present at birth, feeblemindedness was popular among eugenicists as a reference point to unchanging idiocy, imbecility, or, according to H. H. Goddard, the cognitive ability of a moron. Long after the phrase lost any scientific credibility, the phrasings remained popular. In the same way, mental retardation gave way to the more common current usage of intellectual or mental disability, as distinguished from mental illness.

4. Madison Grant, *The Passing of the Race* (New York: Charles Scribner's Sons, 1916); Lothrop Stoddard, *The Rising Tide of Color: The Threat Against White World-Supremacy* (New York: Charles Scribner's Sons, 1920); on Kellogg's "Race Betterment Conferences," see especially Howard Markel, *The Kelloggs: The Battling Brothers of Battle Creek* (New York: Pantheon Books, 2017), 298–321; Brian C. Wilson, *Dr. John Harvey Kellogg and the Religion of Biologic Living* (Bloomington: Indiana University Press, 2014), 133–70.

5. U.S. Department of Commerce, Bureau of the Census, *Insane and Feebleminded in Institutions, 1910* (Washington, D.C.: Government Printing Office, 1910), 183.

6. Table 57, *Eleventh Census of the United States* (1890); *Report of the Commission on the Segregation, Care, and Treatment of Feeble-Minded and Epileptic Persons in the Commonwealth of Pennsylvania* (Harrisburg: Commonwealth of Pennsylvania, 1913), 7; Frazier, *Menace*, 6.

7. Harry Bruinius, *Better for All the World: The Secret History of Forced Sterilization and America's Quest for Racial Purity* (New York: Alfred A. Knopf, 2006), 157–73.

8. Martin W. Barr and E. F. Maloney, *Types of Mental Defectives* (Philadelphia: P. Blackiston's Sons, 1920), 5.

9. "Stimulating Public Interest in the Feeble-Minded," by E. R. Johnstone, address to the National Conference on Charities and Correction, 1916, DNA Learning Center, Cold Spring Harbor Laboaratory, https://dnalc.cshl.edu/view/11404--Stimulating-Public-Interest-in-the-Feeble-Minded-by-E-R-Johnstone-address-to-the-National-Conferenceof-Charities-and-Correction-1916-.html.

10. Joseph S. Neff et al., *The Degenerate Children of Feeble-Minded Women* (Philadelphia: Department of Public Health and Charities, 1910), 5.

11. Charles H. Frazier, "This Generation and the Next in Relation to Mental Defect," in *University Lectures Delivered by Members of the Faculty* (Philadelphia: University of Pennsylvania 1917), 286–93.

12. Barr and Maloney, *Types of Mental Defectives*, 4.

13. Martin W. Barr, "The Imperative Call of Our Present to Our Future," *Journal of Psycho-Asthenics* 7 (September 1902): 5.

14. Thomas C. Leonard, *Illiberal Reformers: Race, Eugenics, and American Economics in the Progressive Era* (Princeton: Princeton University Press, 2016), 54–74.

15. Daniel J. Kevles, *In the Name of Eugenics: Genetics and the Uses of Human Heredity* (Cambridge: Harvard University Press, 1985); Alison Bashford and Philippa Levine, eds., *The Oxford Handbook of the History of Eugenics* (New York: Oxford University Press, 2010); Christine Rosen, *Preaching Eugenics: Religious Leaders and the American Eugenics Movement* (New York: Oxford University Press, 2004); Mark Haller, *Eugenics: Hereditarian Attitudes in American Thought* (New Brunswick: Rutgers University Press, 1963).

16. Adam Cohen, *Imbeciles: The Supreme Court, American Eugenics, and the Sterilization of Carrie Buck* (New York: Penguin Random House, 2016); Thomas C. Leonard, *Illiberal Reformers*, 89–141.

17. Bell quoted in James W. Trent Jr., *The Manliest Man: Samuel G. Howe and the Contours of Nineteenth-Century American Reform* (Amherst: University of Massachusetts Press, 2012), 191.

18. Theodore M. Porter, *Genetics in the Madhouse: The Unknown History of Human Heredity* (Princeton: Princeton University Press, 2018), 16–64.

19. Galton memoirs quoted in Bashford and Levine, *Oxford Handbook*, 5.

20. "Editorial and Other Notes," *Eugenics Review* 2 (July 1909): 65–66.

21. Nicholas Wright Gillman, *A Life of Sir Francis Galton* (New York: Oxford University Press, 2001), 216.

22. Influential family studies included Henry H. Goddard's *The Kallikak Family* (New York: Macmillan, 1912); Richard Dugdale, *The Jukes: A Study in Crime, Pauperism, Disease, and Heredity* (New York: New York Prison Association, 1877).

23. Laughlin quoted in Harry Bruinius, *Better for All the World: The Secret History of Forced Sterilization and America's Quest for Racial Purity* (New York: Alfred A. Knopf, 2006), 212.

24. Harry Laughlin, *The Legal, Legislative, and Administrative Aspects of Sterilization*, Eugenics Record Office Bulletin 10 B (Cold Spring Harbor, N.Y., 1914), 7.

25. J. Ewing Mears, "The Value of Surgical Procedures in the Solution of the Problem of Race Betterment," Box 1, J. Ewing Mears Papers 1877–1979, Jefferson Medical College, Philadelphia; Paul Lombardo, "When Harvard Said No to Eugenics: The J. Ewing Mears Bequest, 1927," *Perspectives in Biology and Medicine* 57 (2014): 374–92. Martin W. Barr, M.D., "Moral Paranoia," in *Proceedings of the Association of Medical Officers of American Institutions for Idiotic and Feeble-minded Persons (New Haven 1895)* (Faribault, Minn.: Institute

for Defectives, 1895), 522–31.; A. W. Wilmarth, "Presidential Address," in *Proceedings of the Association of Medical Officers of American Institutions for Idiotic and Feeble-minded Persons* (Faribault, Minn.: AMOAIIFMP, 1895), 515–21.

26. Henry Friedlander, *The Origins of Nazi Genocide: From Euthanasia to the Final Solution* (Chapel Hill: University of North Carolina Press, 1995), 23–61; Claudia Koonz, *The Nazi Conscience* (Cambridge: Harvard University Press, 2003), 163–89. See Friedlander's essay, "The Exclusion and Murder of the Disabled," in *Social Outsiders in Nazi Germany*, ed. Robert Gellately and Nathan Stoltzfus (Princeton: Princeton University Press, 2001), 145–64. Per Haave, "Sterilization Under the Swastika: the Case of Norway," *International Journal of Mental Health* 36 (Spring 2007): 45–57; Gunnar Broberg and Nills Roll-Hansen, eds., *Eugenics and the Welfare State: Norway, Sweden, Denmark, and Finland* (East Lansing: Michigan State University Press, 2004); Brigitte Bailer and Juliane Wetzel, *Mass Murder of People with Disabilities and the Holocaust* (Berlin: Metropol-Verlag and International Holocaust Remembrance Alliance, 2019).

27. Julius Paul, "'Three Generations of Imbeciles Are Enough': State Eugenic Sterilization Laws in American Thought and Practice" (Ph.D. diss., Walter Reed Army Institute of Research, 1965), 604–8.

28. 1892 speech quoted in Paul, "Three Generations," 611. It is likely that Kerlin performed his first sterilization without benefit of statute in 1889, if not earlier. He had championed the procedure for years.

29. Act No. 12 and Veto Message, *Commonwealth of Pennsylvania Vetoes by the Governor, Session of 1905* (Harrisburg: Commonwealth of Pennsylvania, 1905), 24–27.

30. Joseph S. Neff, *Tenth Annual Report of the Department of Public Health and Charities* (Philadelphia: Department of Public Health, 1912), 1–2.

31. David J. Rothman, *The Discovery of the Asylum: Social Order and Disorder in the New Republic* (Boston: Little Brown, 1971); Rothman, *Conscience and Convenience: The Asylum and Its Alternatives in Progressive America* (Boston: Little Brown, 1980); Sarah Wise, *Inconvenient People: Lunacy, Liberty, and the Mad-Doctors in Victorian England* (Berkeley: Counterpoint, 2012).

32. Frazier, *Menace*.

33. George H. Knight, ed., *Care and Treatment of the Feeble-Minded, Being a Report of the Eighth Section of the International Congress of Charities, Corrections, and Philanthropy* (Baltimore: Johns Hopkins University Press, 1894), 7.

34. W. W. Hawke, MD, quoted in *Public Provision for the Feeble-Minded (a Symposium)* (Philadelphia: Department of Public Health and Charities, 1911), 4–6. Hawke was superintendent of the Warren State Hospital for the Insane in western Pennsylvania.

35. Charles Davenport, "The Origin and Control of Mental Defectiveness," *Popular Science Magazine* 80 (January 1912): 87–90.

36. Edwin Grant Conklin, "The Value of Negative Eugenics," *Journal of Heredity* 6 (December 1915): 541. Published by the American Genetics Association, *Journal of Heredity* was the successor to the *American Breeders' Magazine*.

37. Conklin, "Value of Negative Eugenics," 538–41. Conklin, who would later serve as president of the Philadelphia-based American Philosophical Society, moved from the University of Pennsylvania to Princeton University in 1908, the year Pennhurst opened, to accept Woodrow Wilson's invitation to chair the Biology Department. He attended graduate school at Johns Hopkins University, like Penn, a center for eugenics activities. Conklin appeared on the cover of the July 3, 1939, issue of *Time* magazine.

38. *Laws of the General Assembly of the Commonwealth of Pennsylvania* (Harrisburg: Commonwealth of Pennsylvania, 1903), 446–50.

39. Act No 424, ibid., 446–51.

40. Ruthie-Marie Beckwith, *Disability Servitude: From Peonage to Poverty* (New York: Palgrave Macmillan, 2016), 5–28.

41. *Report of the Commission on the Segregation, Care, and Treatment of Feeble-Minded and Epileptic Persons in the Commonwealth of Pennsylvania* (Harrisburg: Commonwealth of Pennsylvania, 1913), 68.

42. Ibid., 50.

43. Ibid., 50–51.

44. "Three Generations of Imbeciles," in *The Mind and Faith of Justice Holmes: His Speeches, Essays, Letters, and Judicial Opinions* (New York: Modern Library, 1943), 356–59. For context, see Paul A. Lombardo, *Three Generations, No Imbeciles: Eugenics, the Supreme Court, and Buck v. Bell* (Baltimore: Johns Hopkins University Press, 2008).

45. Lombardo, *Three Generations*, 50–53.

46. Marshall's statement is found in a concurring opinion in City of Cleburne v. Cleburne Living Center (1985), in Brief of Amici Curiae in The Board of Trustees of the University of Alabama v. Patricia Garrett and Milton Ash, nos. 99–1240 (United States Supreme Court, 2000), 7–8.

CHAPTER 2

# Living in a World Apart

J. GREGORY PIRMANN

By design, the Pennshurst State School and Hospital was a "world apart," created in the belief that individuals with intellectual disabilities—the so-called "feebleminded"—posed a threat to society and to human progress. Geograhically isolated and off the social grid, so to speak, Pennhurst from the start was a place unto itself—a hulking maze of buildings and grounds detached from the surrounding environment. One of nearly three hundred state institutions around the country, the story of Pennhurst over eight decades of operation includes the story of the more than 10,600 people for whom Pennhurst became *home*. For better or worse, the residents of Pennhurst shared a *lived* experience, and the story of Pennhurst cannot be told without some sense of the individual stories of people who were sent there. They are interwoven within the narrative of the place and its history.

Within Pennhurst's walls there were two divisions: the educational or industrial department and the custodial or asylum department. Even as the population grew from five hundred to more than three thousand, this categorization held firm. The distinction was utilitarian, organized around who was deemed trainable and therefore *useful* for work, and those judged incapable of development and in need of continuous care. (Measureable "improvement" was the word, a classification that even today determines the extent of services required.) Over its eighty years in operation, the pendulum swung from the former—"working patients"—to the latter—"custodial patients," assessed as unable to progress and not in need of educational and social services. In either case, prominent eugenicists in Pennsylvania and elsewhere asserted all came from "tainted stocks" or had been cursed by hereditary defect. Regardless of their abilities, all residents were commonly referred to as "inmates."

Pennhurst was created by an act of the Pennsylvania Legislature on May 15, 1903. Public Law 424 established a commission charged with identifying a "tract of land so located as to be most accessible, by railroad facilities, to the counties of Eastern Pennsylvania." In addition to finding a site for the facility, the commissioners were to develop a plan for an institution and arrange the construction of buildings "of the best design for the construction of such institution, and without expensive architectural adornments or unduly large or costly administrative accommodations."[1]

Along with their charge to the commission, the legislature appropriated funds sufficient to erect a facility for not less than five hundred persons. Following the notion that form follows function, the 1903 law specified that the buildings should be grouped according to the industrial and custodial populations. Furthermore, the institution was to be "entirely and specifically devoted to the reception, detention, care and training of epileptics and of idiotic and feeble-minded persons of either sex . . . [and] shall provide separate classification of the numerous groups embraced under the terms 'epileptics' and 'idiotic' and 'imbecile' or 'feeble-minded.'"[2]

The eugenic imperative could not have been more intentional and explicit. Residents suffering from epilepsy or paralysis were to be apportioned space within the custodial department. Agricultural training, on the other hand, was part of the educational department, and "the employment of the inmates in the care and raising of stock, and the cultivation of small fruits, vegetables, roots, et cetera, shall be made tributary, when possible, to the maintenance of the institution." In other words, those who could labor to profit the institution were expected to do so. Room and board was their reward, with all funds from the sale of agricultural produce and dairy items going directly to the bottom line.

A companion facility to the larger Western Pennsylvania State Institution (which opened in 1897 and is still in operation as Polk

Center), the Eastern Pennsylvania Institution for the Feeble-Minded and Epileptic admitted its first client on November 23, 1908. Several construction phases permitted not only the addition of women but by the 1950s a burgeoning residential population well over three thousand inmates—seven times the initial projected size. The range and diversity of diagnoses was matched by the ethnic and racial diversity of the residents themselves.

Almost as soon as it opened its doors, Pennhurst encountered problems that would persist for nearly its entire history. Buildings were filled (and overcrowded) as quickly as they could be erected. Like other facilities of its kind, there was always a waiting list for admissions and tremendous pressure to take people whose needs were not the same as those for whom the facility was intended. The following excerpt from Superintendent H. M. Carey's June 1, 1910, report to the board of trustees illustrates the nature of the problems afflicting Pennhurst from its opening. Superintendent Carey noted, "During the first eighteen months of the Institution's existence there was considerable confusion as to the class of patients to be admitted, as the general public apparently did not understand the meaning of the terms 'feeble-minded' and 'epileptic.' All sorts and classes of cases have been sent—the violently insane, with homicidal and suicidal tendencies; the maniac, with delusions of persecutions. . . . moral imbeciles, reformatory cases, criminals and so forth." Constant pressure to admit more people assured that just-finished buildings would be used for purposes other than they were designed. From the beginning the forced mixing of different "classes of patients," poor sanitation, insufficient, overworked, and poorly trained staff added to the woes. This litany of problems changed very little over eight decades.[3]

Another critical concern was the persistent lack of state funding. A 1916 report noted that despite the "best efforts of management" to live within its $200 per capita yearly maintenance allocation, actual costs had been $216.50 for the year. The board of trustees hoped that the General Assembly would set the per capita rate at $225.00 annually for the coming year. If properly managed, which meant skimping on a nutritious diet and harsh labor practices, it was possible for Pennhurst ledgers to record a financial profit.

## "Working Patients" Prior to the 1970s

Behind the idyllic veneer of pageants, sports clubs, and assemblies was the world of work. If you were assigned to the educational side of the facility, you might have gone to school. Or, you might have been assigned early on to one of the shops that made the things the facility needed to survive and remain sustainable—mattresses, clothing, furniture, and the like. Once you were deemed old enough, you would be given a job, a job that paid nothing and that could lead to punishment if you refused it. For men, the jobs usually involved heavy physical labor on the farm, on a maintenance and repair crew, in the laundry, in the storerooms, or in the kitchen. You might also be assigned to providing personal care to the less capable men, anywhere where hands were needed to do the work of the institution. Men might change jobs over the years, but the fact that they were required to work never changed. And make no mistake, their labor provided revenue that supported the institution. Critics recognized this as "peonage," or slavery of a different sort.[4]

After their arrival in the 1920s, women were also needed to keep the institution running. Conforming to notions of "true womanhood" and maternal ability, some females were employed in "patient care," feeding, clothing, dressing, and supervising those who could not do so for themselves. They also worked in the kitchens, in the laundry, in the sewing rooms—everywhere that hands were needed to keep the institution afloat. Residents' assigned jobs were "gendered," to use the phrase, and in keeping with social attitudes about appropriate roles.

Like their male counterparts (with whom they had very little, if any, contact—segregation of the sexes was of paramount importance), the women were not paid for their labor. In fact, employees were prohibited from "tipping" or otherwise giving the "working patients" who labored beside them anything in recognition of their contributions. Compulsory labor without adequate compensation cut down on expenses and kept the need for additional outside staff to a minimum. In this regard, Pennhurst was no different from other institutions of its kind.

The "work boys" and "work girls," as they were called, spent long days at their jobs. Many arose before 5:00 a.m. to start their day and were in bed immediately after dinner so they'd be ready to start again the next day. This daily regimen only began to change in the 1960s when new ideas infiltrated the institution and the notion that people might have a life outside of its walls began to be accepted. But most of Pennhurst's people continued to work until the federal courts outlawed "peonage" (defined as unpaid labor that would otherwise be done by a paid employee) in the early 1970s.

A case in point was a resident who shall be called "Abe." Born in Russia in 1904 (four years before Pennhurst opened), Abe's immigrant family abandoned him in 1909. He became the 337th person to enter the facility, having never been given a chance to succeed in the outside world.[5]

In a sense, Abe not only grew up in Pennhurst; he helped build it. Over the decades Abe held many jobs, chiefly assisting the facility's plasterers and stonemasons. The most remarkable thing about Abe's life at Pennhurst, more so than its length or the contributions he made to the facility, was the fact that he seemed among the happiest people there. He seemed always to put forth a cheeful countenance and to greet employees with a resounding "Hello, my friend."

When people began leaving Pennhurst in the 1970s for the new community-based "group homes," Abe's name was put on the list, even though administrators assumed he probably wouldn't be interested in leaving. That all changed when a local TV crew, reporting on the possible closing of Pennhurst, asked to speak with someone who didn't want to leave. They were introduced to Abe and, when the question was asked, Abe surprised a lot of people by saying that he would love to live elsewhere. And so, in 1980, at the age of seventy-five, Abe moved to his new home in Philadelphia. Abe enjoyed a second life in the "real world" well into his nineties.

## The Custodial or Asylum Department

The dual nature of the institution is best illustrated by the following passage, found in a 1943 pamphlet published for an intended audience of "parents and relatives of the children now in the school and on our waiting list, it is hoped that it may likewise prove useful to social and welfare workers throughout the Commonwealth." "Our aim," explained Superintendent James S. Dean, "is to provide a safe and pleasant home and at the same time try to simulate conditions of the outside world as much as possible, especially for those children whom we hope eventually to restore to society with some measure of self-sufficiency. The entire institution is, in fact, quite comparable to a small city with an adjacent farm."[6] However, board reports and promotional literature rarely mentioned the other and more dependent population, and these booklets did not include photographs of the so-called "custodial department"—except for the occasional complaint that the number of people requiring care was becoming more and more of a problem.

From its beginning, Pennhurst had two mandates. Its primary mission was to provide for the "detention, care and training" of the people who would essentially run the facility—the "working patients" who tilled the farm, operated the laundry, assisted the kitchen staff, and, most importantly, but least visibly, to fulfill the insitution's secondary mission by caring for the individuals who could not care for themselves. These were the inmates assigned to the "custodial department."[7] The biennial reports were filled with photographs of the farms, the kitchens, the mattress shop, the printing presses, the woodworking shop, and all of the other areas where people were "trained" for jobs that rarely led to any future other than continued, unpaid employment in Pennhurst.

After extolling this high-minded purpose, the pamphlet goes on to say that "approximately one-third of our patients are paralyzed, helpless and absolutely hopeless for training. For these unfortunates we can render only custodial bed care. In many instances these children could better have been cared for at home and their presence here simply deprives an opportunity for a more hopeful patient on our waiting list. While we therefore discourage the admission of such hopeless cases, every medical and nursing attention is rendered them."[8]

The most astounding aspect of this statement is that it was made publicly in a document designed to explain the "organization, purpose, program and rules and regulations" of the facility. The weight of the dehumanization that allowed Pennhurst to exist in the first place, combined with the notion that the custodial residents were "helpless and hopeless," made life for this part of Pennhurst's population even more tragic and more lethal. At the time that this "information" booklet was printed (1940s), the "patient population" was approximately 2,400 individuals, with an additional 1,500 people on the waiting list. There were 275 employees.

From its opening, and in spite of the problems documented in their own biennial reports, the board regularly petitioned the legislature to add more buildings. In 1912, the trustees noted that "we are aware how the number of degenerates in this Institution has increased; from what large families they come, as a rule; how rapidly applications for admission are coming in; that the reports are practically the same from other sections of the State." Unable to keep pace with the increased demand, Pennhurst trustees professed a corresponding duty "to urge that sterilization be adopted. Many inmates in our own institution, were they sterilized, would be able to leave and would not be a menace to the community, neither would it be possible for them to reproduce their unfortunate kind." The burden on taxpayers reinforced to trustees the wisdom that, 'an ounce of prevention is worth a pound of cure.' We favor the ounce."[9]

Shortly after the end of World War II, the Pennsylvania Department of Welfare published a pamphlet entitled *A Pictorial History of Mental Institutions in Pennsylvania*. The page devoted to Pennhurst included the following: "It is estimated that there are 190,000 mentally defectives in Pennsylvania, ten percent of whom require institutional care, although only five percent currently are receiving such care. This situation contributes in a considerable degree to juvenile delinquency."

Time and again over the decades, Pennhurst's trustees stated their concern about the need to increase the size of the facility and, more importantly, to provide segregated accommodations for women on a recurring basis. Management complained in 1911, and a 1916 report recommended "the consideration of plans for increasing the capacity of the Institution by the erection of a group of cottages exclusively for female inmates, at sufficient distance from the present group to segregate them." A target figure of 1,200 "girls" seemed feasible at only a "comparatively small additional expense." This would effectively double the current population, with little strain on the nearly completed new administration building, power house, laundry, railroad siding, storehouse, the farms, dairy, piggery, and hennery. Said expansion and improvements could meet the physical and training needs of "these unfortunate boys and girls."

Of all of the ideas encompassed in the institution's charter, the creation of a successful and profitable farm labor system was the one that most shaped the interior life of many Pennhurst residents over half a century. As previously noted, the legislative mandate directed that "the process of an agricultural training shall be primarily considered in the educational department; and that the employment of the inmates in the care and raising of stock, and the cultivation of small fruits, vegetables, roots, etcetera, shall be made tributary, when possible, to the maintenance of the institution." Over the years, the more-or-less celebratory reports submitted by the board of trustees contained more information about the success of the farm programs than they did about the lives of the individuals who made those successes possible. Little or nothing was said about peonage or the involuntary servitude of so-called "feeble-minded" men and women who worked the fields for no pay. Nowhere do you find mention of the abuses and neglect that was chronic.

The economics of farm labor and husbandry flourished from the outset. Soon after the first residents were installed in 1908, the cultivation of rich farmlands in Chester County was underway. Trustees reported that "with the necessary farm equipment, proper fertilization and intelligent tillage, the land promises to give a good account of itself." Indeed, it was noted that the farm produced crops worth more than $3,500.00 in the period from June 1, 1909, to October 1, 1910. The 1910–12 biennial report stated that in January 1911 the cattle herd consisted of fifty-eight animals. In the two-year period, the dairy produced nearly five hundred thousand pounds of milk (and more than eight hundred thousand pounds of manure). There is no mention in the report of any of the "inmates" whose labor made this possible.[10]

The farms were eventually phased out, and by the late 1960s only the dairy herd remained at Pennhurst. The herd was sold off after the 1973 United States District Court decision in *Souder v. Brennan* outlawed peonage in publicly operated institutions. "Peonage" (involuntary servitude) was the practice of using the unpaid labor of the individuals living in an institution to operate that institution. In *Souder v. Brennan*, the Court ruled that federal minimum wage and hour guidelines applied when residents of an institution performed labor that would otherwise be performed by a paid employee. The Justices decreed that any residents who worked to maintain the institution where they lived must be paid for the work they performed. With no money available to pay the "working patients," they were simply told to stop working. Not only did income from the farms vanish, the residents lost this semblence of purposeful labor, no matter how restrictive it had been. An added degree of idleness set in very quickly. The *Souder* decision did not mandate equal pay for equal work.[11]

Farm work was not the only employment to which the labor of the "inmates" was dedicated. "Patient care" was the area in which most individuals were required to work, especially as the number of individuals needing care grew. The people of Pennhurst worked everywhere and their labor became essential to maintaining the facility. While the original legislation talked of "training" as one goal for the institution, the real aim was to keep the place running with unpaid labor, minimizing the number of paid employees needed. In some respects, the very survival of the institution depended on the labor of the residents. The scant statistics on employment that are available makes this obivious.

According to the annual reports, by 1930 a total of 192 employees supported 1,247 individuals. The employee to resident ratio was 1:6.5. Twenty-five years later (1955), the resident population had grown to 3,600, with no more than 500 employees. Thus, at its population peak, the ratio of employees to residents stood at 1:7.2. However, the number of children and adults in "custodial care" (as opposed to the "working patient" population) had grown significantly, while the ratio of paid employees to residents had stayed virtually stagnant. One statistic that shows the growing dependence of the facility on the unpaid labor of its residents is found in two separate documents, published thirty years apart.[12]

According to the 1922 board's report, four paid employees supervised forty "working patients" in the laundry. More than eight hundred thousand articles were processed in the laundry that year. By contrast, in 1953 five paid employees oversaw the work of eighty-two "patients" in the newly renovated laundry, a facility that processed more than five million pounds during the year. One additional paid staff member was added in thirty years, while the "working patient" population in the laundry more than doubled.

With one eye on what the trustees referred to as societal "protection," and the other on efficient cost controls, Pennhurst's directors continuously petitioned the legislature for increased funds and facilities improvements. Training, yes, but societal protection at the same time. It should be noted, however, that even those children who attended skill-centered classes in the "school" received a substandard education segregated from their peers on the outside. Between 1918 and 1955, the trustees' reports reiterated that "the number of applications for admission is steadily increasing. We have been able to admit only a small proportion of these applicants, due to our lack of accommodations."[13]

As has already been noted, from the time it first began accepting custodial residents (1908), conditions at Pennhurst were the frequent subject of scrutiny and public concern. Improvements seemed to come only after unwelcome public exposés, and they were short-lived, with conditions reverting back to their previous state. A case in point is the 1930 annual report wherein trustees noted

> a program of general cleanliness and one of exceeding breadth has been entered upon at Pennhurst. It includes not only cleanliness of the individual patient, but also all of the things which come in contact with him, which has necessitated the purchase of more clothing, beds, bedding and furniture, and also the vast quantities of paint, the putting down of new floors, the reconstruction of various wards and service rooms through the tearing down of walls, the purchase of new tables for the dining rooms, and equipment for the kitchen and other things which were done as rapidly as we could with our own labor and with the funds available.

New plumbing and toilet fixtures were ordered for the dormitory wards, and great efforts were made to remove fire hazards.

This same report repeated a now-familiar anthem that worsening overcrowding "has its disagreeable effects in the discipline of an Institution for mental defectives as in other institutions." Even as serious maintenance issues were detailed, the institution's directors advocated for an increase in residential placements. Pressures were especially accute in the "boys'" and "girls'" living spaces and lavatories. Structural changes would have to meet the increased capacity, and the boys' dining hall in particular would have an enlarged space to meet the swelling population. Furthermore, hallways would now accommodate cribs and beds, and cottages were repurposed and interior walls demolished to provide some measure of temporary relief. As had been the case for more than two decades, and would continue for years to come, the priority was additional space at the least expensive cost to the public.

As the decades passed, the population of the facility grew steadily, with large increases following close behind each construction crew. As each new building became ready for occupancy, new residents flooded in, with as many as one hundred individuals admitted in a single month. The "Female Colony," requested by the board in numerous reports, was finally erected in the late 1920s. It was located a mile away from the central cluster of buildings and the male dormitory. This allowed the number of women in residence to grow and remain separated from the male population. The segregation of males and females on separate campuses, with little chance for interaction between the two groups, continued until 1970 when the facility was reorganized under a developmental model.

Coinciding with the name change to Pennhurst State School and Hospital in the 1920s, two of the four upper campus buildings (the aforementioned "Female Colony") were erected, along with a fully equipped hospital and auditorium. Reflecting the Depression-era economy, only one new building (Female Building #3) was added during the 1930s. Plans for another two buildings were scaled back in the 1940s, a concession to wartime material needs. D Building in the main campus and Female Building #4 were finished after the end of the war. These last buildings were the two largest of the "old" buildings.

Over the decades, each generation of buildings was larger than the preceding one; the principle of efficient "warehousing" dictated the building design more than any notion of livability. From 1950 until 1970, there would be no further construction at Pennhurst. Instead, other facilities would be "annexed." One new building was erected in the early 1970s in direct response to sensational news footage about conditions within the institution. But, in the inimitable fashion of bureaucracies, the new building was designed to fit the impulse for "efficiency" that had driven the growth of the facility over the decades.

While the construction of new buildings was halted from 1950 until 1970, Pennhurst's population continued to grow in size. In the mid-1950s, the facility encompassed more than eighty buildings (with seventeen major residential buildings) and over 1,200 acres either owned or leased. Virtually all of this acreage was under cultivation, except for the land on which the buildings stood. The farming was conducted by "patients" under the direction of a handful of paid employees. The growth in size of the physical plant was reflected in the growth of the population. In 1920, the in-house census was 1,200; in 1930, it stood at 1,300 (with an employee complement of 192) and in 1940, it was 2,200. (Remember that, as noted earlier, only one new building was erected in the 1930s. That this "standstill" status was a product of the Depression rather than any change in philosophy is proven by the increase in population, despite the lack of increased space for these extra people.)

By 1950, the in-house census had reached 2,800. It peaked in 1955 with a total of 3,500 persons residing in the facility, with a staff complement of 360 attendants and nurses. Total complement figures for the year are not readily available, but it is certain that the figure was no more than 500 total staff. After 1955, the in-house population began to drop due to the opening of two "Pennhurst Annexes": one at Mount Alto (now the South Mountain Restoration Center) and the other at White Haven in the Pocono Mountains. The successful treatment of tuberculosis in the 1940s made possible the transion to state-operated developmental centers that eased overcrowding at Pennshurst. These annexes eventually housed more than 900 people, all transferred from Pennhurst. The existence of these "annexes" allowed Pennhurst's on-book census to rise to more than 4,100 people, while the actual in-house census at the facility dropped to 3,200.

Pennhurst's superintendent was administratively responsible for the two annexes until 1961, when they were established as free-standing facilities and the clients living there were formally discharged from Pennhurst. The Mount Alto annex population was transferred to what is now the Hamburg Center and became a Restoration Center for geriatric patients. Hamburg Center remains in operation today, still operating in the old sanitarium buildings. In the 1970s an entirely new facility was built to replace the original White Haven structures. White Haven Center continues in operation, serving several hundred people with intellectual disabilities.

Despite these additional facilities, the overcrowding noted since 1911 only grew worse. Visitors, journalists, and especially family advocates noted the deteriorating conditions: chronic understaffing, rudimentary toilet and bathing facilities, and inadequate maintenance of buildings and grounds. Primitive bathrooms and the lack of privacy exacerbated a loss of dignity and basic daily hygiene. The history of Q Building, one of the first residences opened in 1908, illustrates the degree of overcrowding. It was not a large building. Indeed, when modern residential and life-safety standards were finally applied in the 1970s, the building had a listed capacity of sixteen people per floor. Contrast this with the August 1955 census of the building—144 people lived there that month.

Residents of the "custodial department" felt the impact of overcrowded, deteriorating, and unsafe living conditions more than those assigned to the "industrial" program. The burgeoning numbers of custodial "inmates" were literally confined in their wards all of the time, and no physical or occupational therapy was made available. Children were manacled to their cribs and beds—especially those with behavioral problems or severe physical needs—and only rarely removed from their beds. Too frequently, visitors to the dayrooms were assaulted by the sounds, smells, and and images of idle residents who paced the floor aimlessly. Under the guise of puposeful training, so-called "working patients" routinely provided much of the day-to-day personal care.

Amidst enormous public controversy fueled by news media exposés and parental advocacy, in 1970 Pennhurst became one of the first state-operated institutions to reject the custodial, illness model that had been in operation for six decades. In its place, a "developmental model" of treatment was initiated. The most critical change was the belief that all people could learn, all people could grow, and with proper resources all people could experience a better life than Pennhurst provided.

Pennsylvania also became one of the first states in the country to establish a formal system of community residences, operated by private providers and located in neighborhoods, not in a distant countryside. Importantly, these community residences were scaled to the size of a normal family, something Samuel Gridley Howe had advocated more than a century earlier. In many other states, community homes are still, today, sized like mini-institutions.[14] Pennsylvania chose to limit the number of people who could live together to four or less, so that their experience in the "real world" would be real, not simply a smaller version of Pennhurst.

Going hand-in-hand with the changes initiated at Pennhurst in the 1970s and across the Commonwealth was groundbreaking litigation. Prior to the landmark case *Halderman v. Pennhurst*, institutional litigation was focused on "fixing" conditions in the facilities. The Pennhurst case was the first that said that places like it could not be fixed, that no matter what was done, no matter how much money was spent, the life provided in a "world apart" was never going to be the life that people wanted or deserved. Among other outworn and erroneous concepts, the Pennhurst experience disproved the popular notion that some people were "too disabled" to live in the community.

One of the results of the changing social and political attitudes in the 1960s was a new degree of choices made available to some residents. In 1967, Pennhurst was awarded a federal Hospital Improvement Program grant designed to provide specialized supports to individuals with visual impairments. Two of the first beneficiaries were Violet and Leonard, adults who had lived within institutional walls all their lives. Both had severe visual impairments. To carry out the grant program, two "Vision Units"—one for men and the other for women—were opened adjacent to the hospital building annex.

Allowing men and women to live near one another was a radical concept at the time, but this was a time when changes to the old ways of thinking were finally starting to take hold. Given this opportunity, Violet and Leonard became friends. In another sign of the changing times they were both selected to participate in a job placement program and they were eventually both hired to work in the Housekeeping Department of a local hospital. They moved (separately) into their own apartments and their relationship continued as they started their new lives.

Less than a year after she left Pennhurst, Violet became ill and needed to be hospitalized. The counselors assigned to her "case" decided that she should return to Pennhurst because they were concerned about her ability to manage her own health care. Violet would not hear of it, and, as she explained it to me later, she enlisted Leonard to help her stay put. And she also decided that the best way to make sure that she and Leonard would not be separated or returned to Pennhurst was for them to get married. Leonard agreed. Their shared decision was an act of self-determination, to use the new phrase, and devotion to each other. Even though the Pennhurst authorities opposed their marriage, Violet and Leonard became husband and wife in 1971. Here was self-determination in action, a novel concept at the time.

Their marriage lasted more than thirty-five years, and they became mainstays in their community. Leonard died in 2007 and Violet joined him just over a year later. From life in a world apart, they connected with each other in a manner that permitted them, with the right supports, to flourish in the outside world beyond Pennhurst.

## Postscript: An Unprecedented Case Study

In 1979, an advocate named Lou Chapman did something no one had ever done before. Chapman went to live at Pennhurst for forty-eight hours, and she wrote about her experiences in an essay entitled "Living at Pennhurst Center: Observations and Feeling." Not everyone appreciated nor agreed with Chapman's characterization of the interior world, or the unwelcome exposure it brought to institutional life. Her words, however, carried an authenticity born of direct, personal experience with the sights, sounds, and smells of the wards and dayrooms. Furthermore, her role with an advocacy group known as the Pennhurst Human Rights Committee partially prepared her for what she saw.[15] Lou Chapman provided the clearest statement of living conditions at Pennhurst.

At the invitation of Dr. James Hirst, director of psychological services and chief advocate of human rights, representatives of an advocacy group known as the Pennhurst Human Rights Committee were permitted to "live-in" on a ward. Hirst was convinced that such an experience would demonstrated the improvements that had been made in the decade following Bill Baldini's newscast. It was a risky venture.

"I volunteered to participate in the live-in," Chapman explained. "Although I spent a good bit of time 'on grounds' as an advocate," she explained, "I was concerned about my ability to understand what the people who live there really experience. . . . I thought, 'Well, 48 hours isn't very long. I won't go in with any set of expectations, because I doubt if I'll get much out of it in only 48 hours.' I was surprised to discover some of the feelings I did have in that very short period of time. Those feelings had a profound effect on me."[16]

For two days, Chapman lived on a ward with fourteen women classified as severely and profoundly retarded. "I tried to live there as a resident, not to monitor the situation, but to experience it in a feeling and sensory way. However, I did make an effort to integrate myself into the group of women who live there. I ate with them; I slept with them; and I did not leave the ward for 48 hours."

Almost immediately, Chapman noticed the women wore new clothes and white sneakers. "They were glaring like flashlights. A staff person remarked that perhaps I ought to spend time on every ward so that everybody would get new sneakers." She also noticed that the number of staff persons per shift had increased during her stay.

"One of the first things that impressed me was the behavior of these women. It reminded me of the behavior of individuals we call autistic, who have withdrawn from other people. They also had a good many kinds of institutional behaviors with which we are all familiar—pacing, repetitive hand motions, rocking." Chapman concluded the behaviors were an attempt to shut out the environment. "The noise level on the ward was overpowering—the television set was going 24 hours a day, literally, and at certain times the stereo was competing with the television." Unable to leave the ward, residents seemed to escape by retreating into themselves. There was little structured interaction among the residents. Metal plate mirrors in the common bathroom gave women a distorted self-image not unlike the distorted world around them.

The residents were similarly dressed and all had the same bowl-cut haircut with bangs. It was the institutional look found in many facilities. "The only objects available for our entertainment in the dayroom were children's stuffed animals, push toys, balls, coloring books, and some women's magazines. The people who live there range in age from twenty-five to fifty-five. Not surprisingly, some of the staff treated the women like little children, referring to them as "my girls," "How's my little Gerry today?" or "the MRs."

"The staff was most sensitive to my privacy," Chapman remembered. They said, "Now, when you want to take a shower, you be sure and tell the staff." So the staff cleared out when I wanted to take a shower. I was asked if I wanted a privacy screen around my bed. (I didn't.) But I saw a very different attitude toward the people who live there. In fact, on the second shift, there were three men doing all the toileting and showering of the women. I had trouble just physically being there during this process seeing these men with their hands all over the women, during the showering and toweling. To me, it was terribly dehumanizing."

The system of compliance present from the start was still very much in place, and Chapman thought attitudes toward the residents had changed very little. "It's obvious to me that while these ladies are labeled severely and profoundly retarded, they've got a lot of potential if the environment were different, if they were given individual one-on-one programming, and if the staff were properly trained. I know they could progress beyond where they are right now."

Long stretches of idleness perpetuated the self-stim behaviors, and the aggressions residents often displayed toward staff and toward each other—especially in the overcrowded dayrooms. "There are enormous amounts of time when nothing is done. The high point of the day is when someone smears herself with feces; she then gets a one-on-one shower with talcum powder added for good measure and returns to doing nothing." Much like Baldini had recorded in 1968, "some of these women have not given up inventing ways for attention, [but] many others show complete resignation. . . . The feeling I had was of absolute lethargy. I could see this feeling transmitted to the staff, as well. The lack of stimulation was so great that it became an effort to get off the chair and move." "You are so totally isolated from the outside world," Chapman concluded, "that you feel there is no outside world—that the sum total of existence is contained in this room."

As Lou Chapman's words powerfully reiterate, life in an institutional setting was relentlessly monotonous for the vast majority of residents. Grueling labor conditions existed for those who were able to work and thus "earn their keep." A lack of day programming, little supervision or direction, and the sheer absence of meaningful supports and services shaped the diminished quality of life. Perhaps most disturbing in the emphasis on control and compliance was the utter lack of freedom and the continuous disregard for even a modicum of human dignity. There was no privacy, and the specter of physical and emotional neglect and abuse cast a long and unsettling shadow over the place and its people. Chapman ended her report on everyday life with a sobering question: "Would I want to live there? If the answer is no, then why in the world do we in any way support another human being living there?"

## Notes

1. Act No. 424, *Laws of the General Assembly of the Commonwealth of Pennsylvania* (Harrisburg: Commonwealth of Pennsylvania, 1903), 446–51.
2. Ibid.
3. *Biennial Report of the Pennhurst Board of Trustees* (Pennhurst, 1910). Unless otherwise noted, all institutional data comes from biennial reports of the board of trustees.
4. Ruthie-Marie Beckwith, *Disability Servitude: From Peonage to Poverty* (New York: Palgrave Macmillan, 2016).
5. This personal anecdote is shared by the author, who met "Abe" shortly after the author came to work at Pennhurst in 1969.

6. *Pennhurst State School: Information*, written and edited by James S, Dean, M.D. (Harrisburg: Commonwealth of Pennsylvania Department of Public Welfare, ca. 1943), 1–2.

7. *Laws of the General Assembly of the Commonwealth of Pennsylvania* (1903).

8. Ibid., 7.

9. Published in 1913, the report of a special Commission on the Segregation, *Care and Treatment of the Feeble-Minded and Epileptic Persons*, reinforced long-standing support of sterilization as a social necessity. See *Report of the Commission on the Segregation, Care and Treatment of Feeble-Minded and Epileptic Persons in the Commonwealth of Pennsylvania* (Harrisburg: Commonwealth of Pennsylvania, 1913), 68.

10. J. Gregory Pirmann and the Pennhurst Memorial and Preservation Alliance, "Making It Work," in *Pennhurst State School and Hospital*, Images in America Series (Charleston: Arcadia, 2015), 39–60; Beckwith, *Disability Servitude*, 43–140.

11. "Souder v. Brennan," Univeristy of Michigan Law School Civil Rights Litigation Clearinghouse, https://www.clearinghouse.net/detail.php?id=15215; see also Beckwith, *Disability Servitude*, 1–54.

12. *Biennial Reports*, 1922–1950.

13. *Biennial Reports* (Harrisburg: Commonwealth of Pennsylvania, 1919–1925).

14. James W. Trent, *The Manliest Man: Samuel G. Howe and the Contours of Nineteenth-Century Reform* (Amherst: University of Massachusetts Press, 2012).

15. Lou Chapman, "Living at Pennhurst Center: Observations and Feelings," (unpublished) October 1979, http://www.elpeecho.com/pennhurst/PDF/LouChapmanReport/LouChapmanReport.pdf.

16. Unless otherwise noted, all quotations are from Chapman, "Living at Pennhurst."

CHAPTER 3

# The Veil of Secrecy

## *A Legacy of Exploitation and Abuse*

JAMES W. CONROY AND DENNIS B. DOWNEY

For Terri Lee Halderman and Nicholas Romeo, and for many other residents over the years, the promise of Pennhurst State School and Hospital became something of a nightmare, filled with everyday horrors and threats to personal safety. Despite physicians' assurances of a benevolent and nurturing environment in which families could be confident their loved ones would be protected, over the decades a persistent pattern of exploitation, neglect, trauma, and physical abuse eroded whatever confidence might have existed. Though legal or medical experts might have advised the admission of a family member to Pennhurst, an acute vulnerability compounded the sense of grief and guilt that was inherent in "putting away" a loved one. So bad were conditions by 1972 that the local *Pottstown Mercury* referred to Pennhurst as the "Shame of Pennsylvania."[1]

For residents like Roland Johnson, an African American adolescent who suffered repeated rapes by older boys, pleas to authorities fell on deaf ears. Whether the perpetrators were staff or fellow residents, the threat of sexual assault was ever-present. Jerome Iannuzzi Jr., who came to Pennhurst at age thirteen, told a reporter he was routinely beaten by employees and shoved into a cold room with no clothes on and left for hours at a time. More than once he was strapped to a chair and underwent electric shock treatment. Iced cold baths were another form of punishment to force compliance. Isolation and solitary confinement were common practices inflicted by the staff on residents who would not acquiesce. "Mentally retarded people have feelings, too," Iannuzzi told an investigator. Public exposure of abuse and unsafe conditions contributed to the federal court consent decree that led to Pennhurst closure in 1987.[2]

Court records and other documents listed at least forty serious injuries to Halderman and more than sixty to Romeo during their years at Pennhurst. When Romeo left Pennhurst in 1983, his torso bore more than fifty fresh welts, many of them apparently inflicted with a toilet bowl brush. In all, the record showed, Romeo suffered two hundred wounds that were either self-inflicted or at the hands of others. It seemed not to matter that medical professionals had custodial responsibilities of the "inmates." "There was so much animosity toward him [Romeo] it was unbelievable," recalled one aide of his coworkers. "People bragged about getting away with it," said another.[3]

Tragically, a pattern of violence, assault, and outright neglect became commonplace at many of the nearly three hundred public institutions for people with intellectual and developmental disabilities. Neglect and mistreatment cast a long shadow of human indignity at these institutions created to care for society's most defenseless individuals. This was the hard and harsh reality that Samuel Gridley Howe, Dorothea Dix, and other nineteenth-century reformers had warned about generations before. The economy of scale model, and the concentration of more and more residents in confinement, only magnified the problem.

Simply put, a veil of secrecy shrouded a decades-long culture of mistreatment and victimization at Pennhurst. Whether in the farm-dairy-shop labor system that kept residents in a condition of subservience and virtual peonage, or the cycle of surgical and medical experimentation and clinical trials on human subjects, Pennhurst residents were susceptible to one form of exploitation or another.[4]

Most alarming of all was the outright physical violence and psychological trauma many residents experienced at Pennhurst and other state facilities. Once exposed, this pattern led to groundbreaking civil rights litigation and the forced closure of Pennhurst and most institutions for people with intellectual and developmental disabilities—the so-called "mentally retarded" or "feebleminded." Having weathered its own scandals and accusations of malpractice, Polk Center, once the Western State Institution, remains in operation today, as do facilities in Selinsgrove and several other locations.

Ironically, at many institutions across the country, medical staff could be the "first perpetrators," to quote a famous book on medical experimentation.[5] Physicians and other medical personnel played an essential role in assessing who should be sent to Pennhurst and similar custodial centers, and physicians directed the institutional staff that provided hands-on day-to-day treatments. By the 1960s, there were fewer than a dozen trained physicians to supervise care for over three thousand residents at Pennhurst. Nationally, the institutionalized population peaked at over two hundred thousand resident inmates, with chronic overcrowding and understaffing.[6]

Custom, law, and "professional" standards required that medical doctors serve as superintendents of public facilities for individuals with intellectual and developmental disabilities (including epilepsy). For nearly a century, through professional organizations and state medical boards, these same superintendents exerted considerable influence over treatment protocols and public policy, nowhere more so than in Pennsylvania, and they willingly collaborated by making residents available as test subjects. However, the abuse and experimentation that occurred at Pennhurst was remarkably similar to developments across the country.The committal process left residents without the power of consent to treatments. Sometimes physicians did not see the necessity of such consent, believing science served a larger public interest.

Residents became wards of the state, and without oversight they became more susceptible to victimization and a loss of dignity. For much of the twentieth century, a code of silence kept misconduct from public view. So too did the isolation and lack of services, overcrowding, and the absence of external scrutiny. Family visits, if they occurred at all, were kept to a minimum and tightly controlled; parents were not permitted to inspect the actual living quarters in the dormitories. Instead, residents were brought out to meet those who came calling. For many residents and their families, the heartbreaking reality of inadequate care was compounded by physical and sexual assault—the "terror moment," to borrow James Cone's phrase—making Pennhurst and institutions in general a frightening place of custodial incarceration.[7]

One member of the state investigative unit recalled the rape of a teenage girl by an employee who went unpunished, and the habit of staff taking young girls down to the underground tunnels for nefarious purposes. He remembered a resident who "died from eating a State Issue Sock," and another who died from swallowing too much cake. More than once residents who were unsupervised jumped into the top floor laundry shute and fell to their peril on the basement floor.[8] Another famous incident cited in the court records involved a young man who started a fire and died of burn injuries, though the real cause of death was withheld from the family.

All too frequently there were only two or three day staff to provide assistance to as many as eighty patients in a dayroom. Into the 1980s the institutional records document instances of staff members asleep while on duty, and the use of isolation, restraints, and corporal punishment to enforce compliant behaviors. Roland Johnson, who left Pennhurst to become a nationally recognized self-advocate in the disability rights movement, recalled in chilling detail how the overnight hours were the most dangerous time. With a skeletal staff on duty, gangs of older residents would prowl the dormitory wards intent on assaulting and raping defenseless male and female inmates. When Johnson's mother learned of the attacks on her son, she brought the matter up with supervisors, who seemed either powerless or disinterested.[9]

Lou Chapman's human rights report, referred to in the previous chapter, sketched the outlines of petty and pervasive indignities foisted on female residents. Cliff Shaw, the state police officer who conducted an undercover investigation in the fall 1979, remembered staff members pummeling residents with basketballs thrown at their heads and torsos, and one aide named "Smoke" who attacked three residents in the span of three hours. "Most of what I saw was instigated by aides," not residents.[10] Rumors got back to investigators of boxing matches that pitted residents against each other, organized by and for the amusement of the support staff.

In glaring and persuasive detail, federal court filings on behalf of Terri Lee Halderman (1974) and Nicholas Romeo (1982), the accounts of other residents, and documentary news reports like Bill Baldini's groundbreaking five-part *Suffer the Little Children* (1968) contradicted the official utterances (and promotional videos) that Pennhurst was a safe and secure *home*.[11] What became evident was that after more than a half century, whatever commitment to training for a purposeful life outside the institution had existed seemed to have surrendered to a terror-filled regime that contradicted the ethos of compassionate care. Such instances of mistreatment also undermined the physicians' code of "do no harm" to patients.[12]

By the mid-1960s, allegations of abuse, neglect, and medical mistreatment at Pennhurst, Willowbrook, Faribault, Jacksonville (Illinois), Vineland, Polk Center, Sonoma State, and scores of other state-operated facilities for individuals with mental disabilities, prompted a new wave of family, organizational, and self-advocacy. These revelations also led to pioneering litigation in state and federal courts, as in the cases of Halderman and Romeo. (What began as simple efforts to secure services and to reform a corrupted system ended with the closure of scores of public institutions.)

Equally important were the professional assessments from the President's Committee on Mental Retardation, first established in the Kennedy administration. Government reports detailed a legacy of discrimination and custodial "abandonment." Following on the heels of Senator Robert Kennedy's (D-New York) well-publicized 1965 visit to Willowbrook State School—"a snake pit," Kennedy said scornfully—and several other state-run institutions, a photographic essay published in 1966 as *Christmas in Purgatory* presented a public image that resembled a living hell.[13] Critics seized on the images of barely clothed custodial residents wandering aimlessly in spartan corridors and dayrooms, the absence of purposeful activities, prolonged verbal and behavioral outbursts that were unaddressed by staff, and the ever-present odor of human excrement. Similarly, the weight of media reporting at Pennhurst revealed a complex legacy of human indignity that accelerated what attorney David Ferleger termed an "anti-institutional" backlash in public policy and the law.[14]

Was there something in the very nature of Pennhurst and the prevailing model of custodial care that led down a slippery slope to neglect, atrocity, and abuse? Did the terminology of mental *defectives* and moral *imbeciles*, as applied to a whole class of citizens, open the Pandora's box of experimentation and mistreatment? Walter Fernald, a celebrated expert in the field and an early Pennhurst consultant, spoke for many professionals when he wrote in 1912, "The feeble-minded are a parasitic, predatory class, never capable of self-support or caring for themselves."[15] Many professionals accepted H. H. Goddard's (another Pennhurst supporter) causal link between mental and moral defect. Such views lingered long after any diagnostic validity had evaporated.

Or was it simply bad management and woefully inadequate staffing that explains the commonplace cycle of horrors over decades of institutional existence? After all, Pennhurst's population grew from one hundred to more than three thousand residents in the 1960s. Baldini reported in 1968 that there were still nearly three thousand residents on the campus with fewer than a dozen trained physicians; the resident to staff ratio stood at 50:1. However one answers these questions, the realities of human volition and willfulness on the part of the perpetrators cannot be dismissed.

## Experimentation and a Question of Medical Ethics

Two pivotal events helped to establish Pennhurst State School and Hospital as an experimental research site: the 1918 Great Influenza and the onset of World War II.[16] Each contained a public health crisis of staggering proportions and at least indirectly expanded the role of a scientific research culture in perpetuating underlying patterns of abuse and medical mistreatment at state institutions. In the larger context of serving science and the "public good," state institutions for the mentally disabled became investigative laboratories and experimentation stations for novel surgical and therapeutic treatments on unsuspecting residents who had been deprived of their rights to liberty and consent. These procedures included sexual sterilization, autopsies, cranial lobotomies, electro-convulsive therapy (shock treatment), x-rays, and radiation exposure. When new vaccines and psychotropic drugs needed testing, who better to enlist than residents at state institutions? One of the most sensitive ethical debates among research scientists and institutional superintendents was whether informed consent was required of children and young adults with cognitive disabilities.

Human tissue dissection complemented experimental food supplements and dietary additives, and surgery and dental care without the use of anesthesia or proper pain management were common in many institutions. Pennhurst used improper physical restraints—locked and windowless closets, cages, shackles, solitary confinement, powerful medications—and other forms of sensory deprivation to control residents and assess their responses. It is worth noting that some of these commonplace practices predated the racial hygiene laws and euthanasia clinics in Nazi Germany.

Public facilities for individuals with mental disabilities served medical science and the public interest.[17] From the earliest involuntary surgical sterilizations to more comprehensive government-funded campaigns to combat contagious diseases like malaria, influenza, typhus, meningitis, hepatitis, diphtheria, measles, mumps, and the great polio trials of the 1950s—residents in public institutions played a crucial role in the development of modern immunology and vaccination. In times of war and peace, an alliance of researchers, policymakers (including the military), and pharmaceutical companies worked with institutional superintendents and staff to test new vaccines and compounds on unsuspecting residents. The U.S. Army and the Public Health Service, as well as the forerunner to the current National Institutes of Health, were active proponents of experimentation and vaccine trials using vulnerable institutional populations—at Pennhurst and elsewhere. When the question arose, physician/superintendents concurred with medical researchers that informed consent was ill-advised and even unnecessary to commence drug trials and other therapies.[18]

Research virologists, immunologists, pediatricians, and infectious disease specialists at prestigious universities like the University of Pennsylvania, New York University, the University of Michigan, Johns Hopkins and Princeton Universities, and the University of Pittsburgh routinely worked with staff physicians in a veritable conspiracy of silence that shrouded medical research from public scrutiny. Such research only compounded a legacy of distrust that was part of institutional life. Pennhurst is a case in point, but by no means was it unique.

Pennhurst's geographic proximity to Philadelphia and its medical schools, and its close connection to the city's public health establishment, helped to forge an essential relationship with the research scientists. This was especially true for the University of Pennsylvania School of Medicine and Jefferson Medical College, where a connection had been created prior to the Great Influenza pandemic of 1918. (The same can be said of Staten Island's Willowbrook State School and New York University, the University of Pittsburgh and nearby Polk State School and Hospital, and the University of Michigan and neighboring institutions like the Ypsilanti Hospital.)

Joseph S. Neff and Samuel Dixon served, respectively, as Philadelphia director of public health and Pennsylvania commissioner of public health. Drs. Isaac Kerlin, Martin W. Barr, and G. Stanley Woodward were educated at UPenn. Local surgeon and race betterment apostle J. Ewing Mears taught for years at Jefferson. Neff did his undergraduate work at UPenn and then matriculated to Jefferson, where he also served on the clinical faculty before moving into community health. Charles H. Frazier, of course, was dean of the UPenn School of Medicine when Pennhurst opened in 1908. Though a biologist by training, E. G. Conklin maintained close ties to the medical community through his work at the American Philosophical Society.

No one played a more crucial role in forging ties between Pennhurst and medical research than UPenn's Joseph Stokes Jr., MD. That relationship was firmly established by the late 1930s and continued uninterrupted for a quarter century. Scion of generations of prominent Philadelphia doctors, Stokes spent almost the entirety of his professional career at UPenn and its Children's Hospital of Philadelphia (CHOP). Among his many accomplishments, Stokes built a world-class hospital and clinical research lab at CHOP. By the late 1930s Stokes served as chief of Pediatric Services and was actively engaged in public health and immunological research, often in collaboration with Werner and Gertrude Henle, refugee scientists who had fled Nazi Germany in 1936. In another moment of irony, just as Henle departed the University of Heidelberg and the summer Olympics opened in Berlin, American eugenicist Harry Laughlin, the individual most responsible for crafting a model sterilization law, received an Honorary Doctor of Medicine degree from Henle's alma mater.

As fears of a second world war swept across the country in the late 1930s, and throughout the United States government, Joseph Stokes played an increasingly important leadership role in government-funded medical research. It did not hurt his cause that Stokes enjoyed a personal friendship with Secretary of War Henry Stimson, who enthusiastically endorsed military-funded medical research. Stokes worked with the American Epidemiological Board, the U.S. Army's Committee on Medical Research, and what would become the National Science Foundation. Not only was he a beneficiary of government, corporate, and private foundation grants for research on infectious diseases, Stokes influenced who else received such largesse. Perhaps most significantly, Stokes led research teams developing vaccines against influenza, measles, and hepatitis. His collaborations with colleagues like Werner and Gertrude Henle vaulted the University of Pennsylvania Medical School to the forefront of immunological and pharmaceutical investigation during and after World War II. All three took an interest in curing infantile paralysis (polio).

Stokes, Henle, and other university researchers (Saul Krugman, Albert Sabin, and Jonas Salk to name a few) relied on the willing cooperation of institutional staff to make custodial residents available for clinical testing. In the competition for cures, this was standard practice at Pennhurst, Willowbrook, and elsewhere. No one would deny that influenza, malaria, viral hepatitis, measles, mumps, polio, and other illnesses posed a public health risk to children and adults. What was questioned at the time, and ever since, was the suitability of injecting active viruses into otherwise healthy individuals—especially young children—without their expressed consent.

Institutional superintendents were complicit in the research and in testing vaccines on children, some of whom became gravely ill or died from mercury poisoning and other serum-based impurities. A cottage industry of medical publications documented the trial-and-error attempts to develop vaccines by using children as human test subjects at Pennhurst and elsewhere. By the late 1930s a formidable alliance of public health researchers, government policymakers, and pharmaceutical companies defined a national agenda to develop vaccines to combat infectious disease with clinical trials at institutions like Pennhurst and Polk, Willowbrook in New York, and Forest Haven and Rosewood near Baltimore. The Public Health Service's better-known Tuskegee Syphilis Experiments in Alabama, and the polio vaccine trials conducted at Polk and state hospitals near Pittsburgh and in Ann Arbor and Ypsilanti, Michigan, were part of the campaign. So too were the now infamous Willowbrook hepatitis studies that Dr. Saul Krugman and NYU colleagues conducted on unsuspecting Willowbrook residents.

After several years of initial study and with the costs associated with using living animals (monkeys) on the rise, in June 1941 Joseph Stokes and Pennhurst's supervising physician James S. Dean exchanged a series of letters regarding access to residents for clinical trials. Stokes acknowledged inoculations against influenza and measles were already underway at local orphanages and hospitals, and he was cooperating with a Chicago team. Unlike prisons, orphanages, and other mental health facilities, Stokes wrote, "I do not believe at Pennhurst consent would be necessary but we would be glad to accede to whatever your judgement may be on this." What went unsaid was the shared belief that the residents themselves need not consent to experimentation.[19] Concerned such testing "might possibly jeopardize the health of the patients or which might subject the institution to criticism," Dean recommended parental permission in some form. Dean seemed more troubled with liability and public scandal than issues of medical ethics. For his part, Stokes accepted the decision but left it to the institutional staff to inform parents and obtain their approval.

Under Stokes and Henle's guidance during and after World War II, hundreds of Pennhurst children and adults became human test subjects exposed to live viruses. Even as the 1947 Nuremberg Code governing medical research insisted on (a) "voluntary consent of the human subject," (b) "the free power of choice," and (c) the "duty and responsibility" of the researcher to assure proper consent, Pennhurst's human subject trials continued.[20] Throughout the 1940s and 1950s, federal and corporate grants supported Stokes and his colleagues who conducted vaccine research at Pennhurst and at institutions in New Jersey. Control groups were inoculated with both live viruses and test vaccines for influenza, hepatitis A and B, and then measles and the mumps. In one instance at Pennhurst several hundred residents were injected with live influenza vaccine with a mineral oil base. Many developed large nodules at the injection site that persisted for up to eighteen months. In other tests, some children experienced mercury poisoning when inoculated with experimental vaccines. Between 1943 and 1946, Stokes and the University of Pennsylvania received nearly $300,000 in military funding for infectious epidemic research.[21] In his official memoir of wartime experiences, Stokes admitted that due to their efforts "the lives of thousands of GI's were probably saved as a result." Despite the wealth of research conducted at Pennhurst, in 1957 an influenza outbreak at the institution killed scores of children and sickened hundreds more.[22] Medical progress was achieved, but at what cost?

Through the School of Medicine, Penn's Children's Hospital, and the affiliated Wistar Institute, human subject research continued into the 1960s. Pharmaceutical company grants—Merck, Wyeth, Pfizer, and Lederle Laboratories were among the major contributors—helped sustain continuous research at Pennhurst and other state institutions in Pennsylvania, New Jersey, and throughout the country; medical personnel willingly cooperated. By the mid-1950s polio (infantile paralysis) gave added urgency to the medical crusade to develop new compounds and therapies.[23]

In 1952 Dr. Hilary Koprowski, who had ties to UPenn and Wistar, stirred controversy for supplementing chocolate milk with a live polio vaccine consumed by residents at Sonoma State School. The same year, University of Pittsburgh virologist Jonas Salk conducted similar experiments at Polk State School and Hospital in western Pennsylvania. As David Rothman has pointed out, access to institutional populations made securing funding for large clinical trials all the easier.

By February 1973, when Pat Clapp and other officials of the Pennsylvania Association of Retarded Citizens (ARC) learned that medical abuses—experimentation without the informed consent of the subjects—were occurring at state institutions; testing at Pennhurst had been ongoing for four decades. What prompted Clapp and other parents to take action was one mother's report that her child had been a "guinea pig" in Dr. Robert Weibel's live virus meningitis trials at the Hamburg State School and Hospital near Reading. (Parents had been informed erroneously that the state ARC endorsed such experiments.)

"I was appalled," she said and almost immediately contacted national ARC president Eleanor Elkin. Clapp confronted Weibel, a noted University of Pennsylvania pediatrician, and learned that other institutions and university researchers were equally culpable. She dismissed Weibel's claim that the children would be "making a contribution to society." Though researchers like Stokes, Henle, and Weibel had deflected accusations of unethical behavior, the media reaction to this new round of reports persuaded state officials to declare a moratorium on medical experimentation and testing at Pennsylvania's custodial institutions.[24]

The veil of secrecy that hid medical experimentation from public scrutiny extended to the equally troublesome pattern of verbal and physical abuse and the intimidation of residents. Revelations of ongoing neglect, mistreatment, and violence, which many outsiders saw for the first time in Baldini's 1968 broadcast, coincided with the Commonwealth of Pennsylvania's moratorium on nonconsensual experimentation on residents at all state institutions. These revelations coincided with several federal lawsuits that undermined the entire architecture of custodial care in Pennsylvania and across the nation. Polk, Willowbrook, Jacksonville (Illinois), west to Sonoma State School in California, the complaints were remarkably similar.

"The typical scene on entering a ward," attorney David Ferleger remembered, "was residents, many of them naked, lying on the floor and in the corners, on benches, doing absolutely nothing. . . . The smell was just overpowering."[25] The same year (1974) Nicholas Romeo arrived at Pennhurst, Ferleger filed a lawsuit on behalf of another resident who had suffered outrageous abuse: Terri Lee Halderman. Affidavits in each proceeding documented the degree of neglect and abuse while shattering the veneer of compassionate custodial care.

The 1979 undercover investigations of staff abuse would lead to seven indictments of Pennhurst employees, with six convictions for criminal assault. This prompted a federal investigation of conditions at Pennhurst.[26]

There is ample evidence of the degree of injury, including resident-on-resident violence, staff assaults and rape, and self-inflicted violence. Internal reports and reports to the Pennsylvania Department of Public Welfare detail the range of dereliction of duties, from petty offenses to persistent patterns of misconduct that jeopardized residents' safety—anything from falling asleep on the job to leaving children unattended in their cribs and beds for long periods of time. Reports included patient deaths by injury or suicide, beatings, unspecified "unethical behavior," cursing and fighting, and even staff who were inebriated when they showed up for work.[27]

A common thread was the lack of direct supervision, something the state police report noted, and the possibilities that with better care and treatment many serious injuries could have been avoided. With a ratio of fifty residents to one or two dayroom staff on most wards (and fewer staff overnight), the threats to personal safety and security were ever-present. For example, in January 1977 there were 833 minor and twenty-five major injuries reported. Rape, physical violence, beatings, and assaults were the commonplace causes, whether perpetrated by a resident or staff member or as the result of an "accident." Accidents included loss of teeth, a resident being blinded, and hundreds of broken limbs and head injuries. All required hospitalization in the infirmary. Children who were unable or unwilling to stop biting had their teeth pulled out without benefit of Novocain or other pain medication. Add to this what outside observers assessed to be less than "minimal professional standards of cleanliness" and inattention to personal hygiene needs, and it should be no surprise that the spread of contagious disease and infections of one kind or another was an ever-present threat.[28]

In this climate of fear, intimidation, neglect, and abuse, many residents regressed in their verbal and occupational skills, muscles atrophied without proper therapy and exercise, and some remained heavily medicated to dampen down outbursts and behavioral oddities.

At least until the late 1970s, educational and social services were not available, nor was a proper regimen of diet and exercise. Incidents of mistreatment and malpractice that surfaced at Polk State School and the Hamburg Center were equally egregious.

The experiences of Terri Halderman and Nicholas Romeo, both plaintiffs in legal actions that helped to establish a constitutional right to education and services in the "least restrictive" environment, serve to illustrate the everyday horrors that plagued many Pennhurst residents in its heyday. Furthermore, their cases, known respectively as *Halderman v. Pennhurst State School and Hospital* and *Romeo v. Youngberg,* persuaded the federal judiciary to compel the state to create new safeguards for residents who were victimized by each other, by staff, and by the institutional system itself. As is explained elsewhere, these cases transformed American constitutional law on the basis of equal protection, due process, and the prohibition against cruel and unusual punishment. The suits also addressed the lack of civil liberties afforded institutionalized wards of the state. For Terri Halderman and Nick Romeo, as for many other residents with severe or profound mental disability, the everyday horrors of overcrowding, inadequate supervision and services, and a general lack of engagement amounted to maltreatment that they were not defended against.[29]

Like Bill Baldini's *Suffer the Little Children* exposé, court litigation of behalf of Terri Lee Halderman, Nicholas Romeo, and other Pennhurst residents exposed the harsh and inhumane conditions present at Pennhurst in the 1970s. As will be examined in detail elsewhere, both Halderman and Romeo were judged to be severely and profoundly disabled based on cognitive measurements. Supported by a battery of attorneys that included David Ferleger, Thomas Gilhool, Judith Gran, and Frank Laski, the separate challenges wound their way through a maze of state and federal courts before ending up before the United States Supreme Court in 1981 and 1982, respectively. At issue was the obligation of the state to provide adequate personal security, meaningful training, and freedom from cruel and unusual punishment. It raised fundamental constitutional questions about the rights and protections due citizens with intellectual and development disabilities, whether their incarceration was voluntary or not.

Lest one fall into the "easy out" of assuming that these things happened only to a few, it is worth pointing out that decades after Pennhurst closed in 1987 the members of the advocacy group Speaking for Ourselves were still in the process of finally admitting that they had been physically, sexually, and psychologically abused at Pennhurst. A therapist continues to counsel victims and help the members recover from their abuse and post-trauma troubles. Many of the friends, advocates, advisors, and facilitators of Speaking for Ourselves have been interviewed in the course of working on this book. When their reflections are all put together, it becomes clear that abuse was the norm, not the exception, at the institution.[30]

It is also important to keep in mind that most of the members of Speaking for Ourselves were not able to communicate. Just over half of the people who lived at Pennhurst in 1978 did not use verbal language. Their full stories will never be told. Chillingly, people who cannot speak are among the most victimized—because they cannot testify against their abusers.[31]

Perhaps the most telling way to conclude this chapter on experimentation and abuse is to quote the words of one parent that were included in the original complaint filed in federal court in 1974. The passage captures the clear sense of the everyday horrors that existed behind a veil of secrecy at public institutions in those days:

> Plaintiff Robert Hight, born in 1965, was admitted to Pennhurst in September, 1974. He was placed on a ward with forty-five other residents. His parents visited him two and one-half weeks after his admission and found that he was badly bruised, his mouth was cut, he was heavily drugged and did not recognize his mother. On this visit, the Hights observed twenty-five residents walking the ward naked, others were only partially dressed. During this short period of time, Robert had lost skills that he had possessed prior to his admission. The Hights promptly removed Robert from the institution, Mrs. Hight commenting that she "wouldn't leave a dog in conditions like that."[32]

## Notes

1. "Pennhurst: The Shame of Pennsylvania," *Pottstown Mercury*, August 8, 1972, 1.

2. Roland Johnson, *Lost in a Desert World: An Autobiography (as Told to Karl Williams)* (Philadelphia: Speaking for Ourselves, 1994); "He lived a Pennhurst horror story," clipping file, Speaking for Ourselves Collection, Elwyn.

3. John Woestendier, "The Deinstitutionalization of Nicholas Romeo," *Philadelphia Inquirer Magazine*, May 27, 1984, 18–24, 30; Halderman v. Pennhurst State School and Hospital, 446 F. Supp. 1295 (E.D. Pa. 1977) at 1308 and 1318.

4. Ruthie-Marie Beckwith, *Disability Servitude: From Peonage to Poverty* (New York: Palgrave Macmillan, 2016), 1–54; Sidney Halpern, *Lesser Harms: The Morality of Risk in Medical Research* (Chicago: University of Chicago Press, 2004); Henry K. Beecher, "Ethics and Clinical Research," *New England Journal of Medicine* 274, no. 24 (June 16, 1966): 367–72.

5. Wendy Lower, *Hitler's Furies: German Women in the Nazi Killing Fields* (Boston: Houghton Mifflin, 2013); see also Robert Jay Lifton, *The Nazi Doctors: Medical Killing and the Psychology of Genocide* (New York: Basic Books, 1986).

6. Beckwith, *Disability Servitude*, 24.

7. James Cone, *The Cross and the Lynching Tree* (Maryknoll, N.Y.: Orbis Books, 2011), 202.

8. Cliff Shaw, email message to Dennis B. Downey, March 28, 2019.

9. Roland Johnson, *Lost in a Desert World.*

10. Cliff Shaw, interview by the editors, Paradise, Pennsylvania, September 25, 2018.

11. "Halderman v. Pennhurst" Disability Justice, http://disabilityjustice.org/halderman-v-pennhurst-state-school-hospital. This website contains a synopsis of relevant court decisions, as well as articles and interviews with David Ferleger, Thomas Gilhool, Judith Gran, James Conroy, and others involved in groundbreaking litigation and research.

12. David J. Rothman, *Strangers at the Bedside: A History of How Law and Bioethics Transformed Medical Decision-Making* (New York: Basic Books, 1991), 37–39.

13. Burton Blatt and Fred Kaplan, *Christmas in Purgatory: A Photographic Essay on Mental Retardation* (1966; Syracuse: Human Policy Press, 1974). A follow-up exposé was published in 1979. President's Committee on Mental Retardation, *Mental Retardation Past and Present*, MR 77 (Washington, D.C.: Government Printing Office, 1977); John H. Bohrer, *The Revolution of Robert Kennedy: From Power to Protest After JFK* (New York: Bloomsbury Press, 2017), 211.

14. David Ferleger and Penelope A. Boyd, "Anti-Institutionalization: The Promise of the Pennhurst Case," in "Symposium: Mentally Retarded People and the Law," *Stanford Law Review* 31, no. 4 (April 1979): 717–52. Isaac N. Kerlin, the superintendent at nearby Elwyn and the leading practitioner/administrator until his death in 1893, invented the phrase "moral imbecile" to explain individuals with a mental disorder who "lack the moral control over the lower propensities." Isaac N. Kerlin and John M. Broomall, *Moral Imbecility* (Philadelphia: Lippincott, 1889), 4. In his classification scheme, mental and moral instability went hand in hand.

15. W. E. Fernald, "The Burden of Feeblemindedness," *Journal of Psycho Asthenics* 18 (1912): 90–98.

16. John M. Barry, *The Great Influenza: The Story of the Deadliest Pandemic in History* (New York: Penguin Books, 2005). An estimated fifty to one hundred million people worldwide, and more than six hundred thousand Americans, died during the 1918–19 outbreak. Philadelphia's decision not to cancel a Liberty Parade contributed to the virus's rapid dissemination throughout the city.

17. David J. Rothman, "Ethics and Human Experimentation: Henry Beecher Revisited," *New England Journal of Medicine* 5 (November 1987): 1354–60.

18. For an introduction to American human subject research, see Susan E. Lederer, *Subjected to Science: Human Experimentation in America Before the Second World War* (Baltimore: Johns Hopkins University Press, 1997); Harriet A. Washington, *Medical Apartheid: The Dark History of Medical Experimentation on Black Americans from Colonial Times to the Present* (2006; New York: Doubleday, 2008), esp. chaps. 8–10, 13; Susan M. Reverby, *Examining Tuskegee: The Infamous Syphilis Study and Its Legacy* (Chapel Hill: University of North Carolina Press, 2009); Allen M. Hornblum, Judith L. Newman, and Gregory J. Dober, *Against Their Will: The Secret History of Medical Experimentation on Children in Cold War America* (New York: Palgrave Macmillan, 2013).

19. Stokes quoted in Sidney Halpern, *Lesser Harms: The Morality of Risk in Medical Research* (Chicago: University of Chicago Press, 2004), 93–100, cf. 24, 25.

20. Promulgated in response to the criminal prosecution of Nazi physicians and their wartime experimentation on people with disabilities and other groups, the Nuremberg Code established international norms in medical ethics and human subject research. See "Nuremburg Code" United States Holocaust Memorial Museum, https://www.ushmm.org/information/exhibitions/online-exhibitions/special-focus/doctors-trial/nuremberg-code#Permissible.

21. Joseph Stokes Jr. Papers, American Philosophical Society, Philadelphia, PA., Series 3, box 148; "1943 Annual Report, Commission on Measles and Mumps," U.S. Army Medical Department, Office of Medical History, http://history.amedd.army.mil/booksdocs/historiesofcomsn/section1.html; Rothman, *Strangers at the Bedside*, 37–38.

22. "The Armed Forces Epidemiological Board: Its First Fifty Years; The Appendicies, Appendix 2. A Memoir by Joseph Stokes, Jr. M.D." U.S. Army Medical Department Office of Medical History, Books and Documents, http://history.amedd.army.mil/booksdocs/itsfirst50yrs/appendices.html.

23. Meredith Wadman, *The Vaccine Race: Science, Politics, and the Human Costs of Defeating Disease* (New York: Viking Press, 2017), 19–43, 112–29.

24. Hornblum et al., *Against Their Will*, 81–86; Linda Drummond, *ARC Pennsylvania, Historical Overview: 1949–1990*, http://www.thearcpa.org/resources/historicaldocs.html.

25. John Woestendiek, "The Unwitting Revolutionary of Pennhurst," *Philadelphia Inquirer Magazine*, May 27, 1984, 22.

26. Cliff Shaw interview 2018.

27. Elmer McSurdy, "Personnel Disciplinary Actions Memo," May 6, 1971, http://www.elpeecho.com/pennhurst/PDF/PersonnelDisciplinaryActions/1971-05-06PersonnelDisciplinaryActions.pdf.

28. Excerpt from federal court filing, Halderman v. Pennhurst State School and Hospital, 446 F. Supp. 1295 (E.D. Pa. 1977) at 1308 and 1318, http://www.preservepennhurst.org/default.aspx?pg=36.

29. "Pennhurst State School and Hospital v. Halderman" U.S. Supreme Court Decisions, Legal Information Institute Collection at Cornell Law School, https://www.law.cornell.edu/supremecourt/text/451/1; "Youngberg v. Romeo," U.S. Supreme Court Decisions, Legal Information Institute Collection at Cornell Law School, https://www.law.cornell.edu/supremecourt/text/457/307.

30. Speaking for Ourselves is the organization of people advocating for themselves that grew out of the Pennhurst experience. Its emergence and vision is described in chapter 7.

31. Richard Sobsey, *Violence and Abuse in the Lives of People with Disabilities: The End of Silent Acceptance?* (Baltimore: Paul H. Brookes, 1994).

32. Halderman v. Pennhurst, 1974.

PART 2

# The Power of Advocacy

Part 2 explores the rise and eventual success of organizational and self-advocacy in challenging the institutionalization model. The deteriorating conditions at Pennhurst prompted a wave of public advocacy in the 1960s and 1970s. In the media, in the courts, and in the boardrooms where government policy was shaped, activism prompted a reconsideration of the fundamental tenets of institutionalization. Investigative journalism, constitutional law, and organizational and self-advocacy conspired to launch a disability rights movement modeled on the modern civil rights movement. Though the Commonwealth of Pennsylvania committed millions of dollars to Pennhurst's "improvement," equal protection, due process, and the right to services in the least restrictive environment mandated institutional changes that led ultimately to Pennhurst's closure in 1987. The same was true in many other states.

Terminology and diagnostic therapies changed, as did behavioral theory and public policy. Often those most directly involved in the constitutional struggle had a direct connection to someone who had lived at Pennhurst, or some other institution. In this sense, the personal informed the public campaign for rights, social recognition, and dignity. A fundamental question lingered: were institutionalized citizens better off—was their quality of life improved—once they left places like Pennhurst?

CHAPTER 4

# *Suffer the Little Children*

## *An Oral Remembrance*

BILL BALDINI

In July 1968 television viewers in the greater Philadelphia area were transfixed by an unprecedented broadcast of life within a state institution for children and adults with intellectual and developmental disabilities. Aptly titled *Suffer the Little Children*, the groundbreaking exposé ran over five nights on WCAU, then the local CBS (now NBC) affiliate, revealing for many the squalid and neglectful conditions at Pennhurst State School and Hospital. For Bill Baldini, the young reporter given access to the interior spaces, the experience was life altering, and the documentary garnered national attention. It also had a profound effect on the growing anti-institutionalization movement. To this day, *Suffer the Little Children* is frequently cited as a cataclysmic moment in the disability rights movement. A half century later, Baldini's reporting serves as a reminder of the power of the media to shape public perceptions and make visible the harsh realities of inhumane public policy.

Bill Baldini's personal recollections amount to an oral history of a seminal moment that shattered the complacency of policymakers and the viewing public. What follows is Baldini's personal account of those events. He came to Jim Conroy's office for a recorded interview in late 2014. A detailed transcription of their conversation follows. Only one question was asked of Baldini: How did you get into this?[1]

The truth of the matter is that I was a very young and inexperienced reporter. This is like my first real job. Before that I was a writer of the news, but I'd never reported. I think on a Sunday, I had nothing to do. And the Marriott used to have conferences all the time. So I said to this guy who was on my assignment desk, why don't I just go to the Marriott, see what's going on over there, because we've got nothing happening.

I went to the Marriott, and the Main Line Junior Chamber of Commerce was having a meeting. And they were talking about this place called Pennhurst that they had visited the week before. And this PR man named Jerry Haas came over to me and asked me who I was and I told him and he started telling me about Pennhurst. What they saw. I did not believe him. I thought, "This is a gross exaggeration." At which point I told him, "If one-tenth of what you're telling me is true, I'll do a story on it." And I meant one-tenth. To make a long story short, I figured I couldn't get in there with a camera, so I said, "Why don't you swear me in, as a member of the Junior Chamber of Commerce, and I'll go with you next Sunday as one of you. And I'll see what you're talking about." Which I did.

I was blown away. I could not believe what I was seeing. You know, you go into various wards, and see these people in various states of undress. And you see them sitting in their own feces. You see a thousand flies around. You see people banging their heads, and nobody's stopping them. And the smell was overwhelming.

By the time I finished that little trip, I was in shock. So I told this guy from the Junior Chamber of Commerce, "I'll definitely do a story on this." I've just got to figure out how.

So I went back to work, and I told my boss, who did not believe me. He had the same exact reaction I had. Like the kid's crazy. I was the kid. And I said, "Barry, you've got to trust me." He says, "Well, how are you going to get in there?" and I said, "I am going to go up there, and tell this guy that if he does not allow me in, or whoever the superintendent is, I'm going to stand in front of the gate every day and tell people what I saw inside."

So frankly, that's what happened. I went up the next week with the Junior Chamber of Commerce, who was there to volunteer to investigate and do whatever they could do. And I talked with the superintendent, a fellow named Leopold Potkonski, and I told him, "Doctor, this place is a mess. It's incredible, I've never seen anything like this. Why is it like this?" And he said, "Because we can't get any money," and so on and so forth. And I said, "Well, I'm really from Channel 10, I'm going to stand outside the gates every day and tell people what I saw—unless you let me come in with a camera."

Much to my shock and surprise, he says, "OK." And I'm twenty-six years old. I was like, "What!!??" Okay, this is great, and I went up there. I got the best cameraman we had, the best sound man, and we went up there. And they literally got sick. First day. They were like, "I can't do it." I said, "You have to do it." And fortunately they got into it as much as me, and overcame the shock and surprise, and the smells, and did their job.

Now, once we were there, shooting this stuff, these people who worked there, these attendants, the management, I would say at least half of that staff was ecstatic. Because they knew it was wrong. They just couldn't change the system. "If I speak up, I'm going to lose this job, and it's not the greatest job, but it's the only job I have, and nobody listens to me anyway." And they looked at me like, here's an opportunity that someone from the outside will look at this and try to change it. So they're feeding me information left and right. Without them, I couldn't have done it. They're telling me where to go. I didn't know where to go. Nobody would have known where to go. They told me where to go, and who to see.

And I went there every single day, and when I brought back the first rushes, as we used to call them, management at Channel 10 could not believe what they were seeing. They said, "Well, we've got to put this on the air."

I said, we'll go out to Pennhurst, we'll leave the station at 8:00, get there by 9:00. We were there all day. And then at 5:00 we would leave, bring it back, and at the time it was film, so we had to process the film. Then after you process all this film, I had to look at it. And then I had to write it. And then have it edited. So I'm there—my days were like twenty hours a day. And I wasn't getting any sleep. So I'd go back the next day.

So when we put it on the air for the first time, the response was absolutely incredible. To this day, Channel 10 never got a response like that, for anything it ever did. The five nights were called *Suffer the Little Children*. The title was taken from the famous passage in the Gospel of Mark wherein Jesus exhorts the elders to bring the children to him (Mark 10:14–16).

It was overwhelming. The newspapers jumped in, they wanted a piece of this. They actually saw it so they're sending people, but everybody was way behind us. We were just way ahead. But because we were and the competition came in, I had to produce every day.

Let me give you an example. At the time, the word was that no story would be more than one minute and thirty seconds, maybe one minute and forty-five if it was extraordinary. I'm going on for eight minutes, twelve minutes, fifteen minutes, at the end twenty-seven minutes.

So the bottom line was that we were doing everything day to day. And it got so the pressure to produce was intense, because people were so into this story.

To make a long story short, day after day, we were doing this story, and by Thursday, I hadn't slept for four or five days. I'd been taking these pills, like No-Doz, to the point where I just frankly lost my voice. So that Thursday, I actually shot, edited it, wrote it, but I could not record it because I could not speak.

John Facenda took over for the last night. It probably ended up even better because he was so good at it.

But that's how we got to actually get into Pennhurst. We really kind of strong-armed the people there into feeling that we were their only hope. Which we were. I wasn't lying about that. If we didn't get in, that place would have remained the same. I mean they were getting absolutely nowhere when it came to budgets and money. Nobody cared. Nobody cared at all. And all they did was cut back the budget.

The people there were warehoused. That was my thinking at the time. That these people were being hidden away, warehoused, out in Spring City. Which at the time was in the middle of nowhere. Nobody went to Spring City unless he lived there. And that was Pennhurst, and it was a dumping ground for people—you had your mentally retarded people but you also had mentally ill people there. If you had any type of person they didn't know what to do with, send them to Pennhurst. Just get them out of here. It was terrible. This was 1968.

What happened was, after that, and I told you the response was incredible, CBS decided to send this copy of what we did out to every CBS station. The order was for every CBS news director in every city to find a place like Pennhurst and get in. This was how an affiliate in New York City acquired the idea to investigate conditions at the Willowbrook institution on Staten Island six years later—in 1974—and it became a story that boosted another young newsman's career, Geraldo Rivera.

Lots of people got involved. The Kennedys got involved. They sent me a letter. I'll tell you who else was involved, remember old Richardson Dilworth [then mayor of Philadelphia]? About why aren't these people schooled in public schools? Why aren't they given an equal opportunity for an education? And Richardson Dilworth not only understood it but was honest enough to say, "We just never cared enough."

I wasn't saying that they should be put in public schools, but what I did say, "If you're spending $2,000 on my kid, you should spend $2,000 on the child with disabilities. And give that child an opportunity to be whatever they can become." And he understood that perfectly.

We did at least three follow-ups. I can even remember their names. "No Less Precious" was one. "Lest We Forget" was another. And I did a third, can't remember that name. These were half-hour shows. Those shows are lost, no copies can be found. Never did I dream that it would snowball into what it did. I'm elated, and I've said this to other people. You know, it was my first real story, and I've never done anything that had that kind of impact since. And that's forty-three years of reporting. It's a long time.

## Note

1. In 2003, Bill did another follow-up, for Channel 10 WCAU, called "Pennhurst Revisited," showing how the people who left Pennhurst had flourished. Bill retired officially in 2011, and remains active with many worthy causes, the Pennhurst Memorial and Preservation Alliance among them. The City Council of Philadelphia named March 17 as "Bill Baldini Day" when he hung up his microphone.

CHAPTER 5

# The Rise of Family and Organizational Advocacy

JANET ALBERT-HERMAN AND ELIZABETH COPPOLA

One of the defining moments in the rise of advocacy and its challenge to institutionalization came during World War II. Of the forty thousand men who resisted induction into the armed forces, more than three thousand were assigned to "alternative service" in so-called "camps" within state mental hospitals and schools for people with intellectual disabilities. The greater number of men inducted into alternative service were conscientious objectors opposed to war but willing to perform other duties. Many came from the historic peace churches—Society of Friends (Quakers), Brethren, Mennonite—and their opposition rested on religious grounds.

Directed by the Civilian Public Service, young pacifists like Charles Lord, Warren Sawyer, and Neal Hartman (and some women) found conditions were appalling at Byberry, Norristown, Pennhurst, and Polk, and more than fifty other centers. "I called them hellholes," Sawyer recalled. Conditions were so bad at Pennhurst that the American Friends Service Committee withdrew its support and ceded sponsorship back to the government. With photos in hand, Lord and other conscientious objectors (COs) took their complaints to President Franklin D. Roosevelt, but it was not until after the war that Mrs. Roosevelt took an active interest. In 1946, *Life* magazine published a story accompanied by Charlie Lord's photos that seared the public conscience and the public service program was shut down.[1] Its impact on families and subsequent advocacy efforts is hard to overestimate.

CO accounts of horrific conditions appeared in newspapers and magazines, along with startling photographs of life within state facilities for people with intellectual disabilities.[2] The bulk of the publicity centered on Byberry and other psychiatric hospitals. However, they did observe incidents of abuse, neglect, cruelty, and even alleged murder that occurred at Pennhurst and elsewhere.[3] In 1945 the Mental Hygiene Program's Len Edelstein reported he found at Pennhurst "conditions rather similar to those at Byberry [mental hospital in Philadelphia]—namely lovely grounds, nice façade, but very old wooden buildings, dimly lighted and often pervaded with strong odors. The boys, crammed into day rooms—fed poor looking food on metal trays, are often worked twelve hours per day, seven days a week." Anthony Leeds compared Pennhurst State School and Hospital to a "concentration camp." He especially remembered "U-Cottage, a slave house where they were beaten, had arms tied to steam pipes, and [were] made to provide for all major labor of the institution."[4]

The public revelations offered by wartime conscientious objectors breathed new life into fledgling parent groups across the country. The return of more than 671,000 disabled veterans also influenced public awareness of the impact of disabilities on family life. Films like the award-winning *The Best Years of Our Lives* (1946) dramatized the physical and emotional burdens some returnees carried to homefront repatriation. The picture struck a chord, winning seven Academy Awards, including Best Supporting Actor for Harold Russell for his portrayal of "Homer," who has lost both hands from severe burns in combat. But, in a case of art imitating life, it is clear in the film that the families and loved ones suffered along with each of the four returning vets.

With the growth in scientific research and advocacy, parents found that they could sustain and improve the lives of their veteran sons by demanding assistance and opportunities.[5] Publicized awareness of the mistreatment of those living in institutions, as well as medical breakthroughs, also gave parents of children with disabilities new hope for their postwar growing families. The realities of poor care and inadequate staff training, abuse, overcrowding, and long waiting lists undermined faith in public institutions across the country, and at Pennhurst.

The post–World War II organizational efforts of parents created a broad national advocacy network dedicated to improving conditions and services available in either an institutional or community setting. Their courage in protecting their children laid the foundation for a much larger and more powerful disability advocacy organization in America. Eventually their efforts led to the movement for deinstitutionalization and a return to the mainstream, with all the possibilities and uncertainties inherent in the new provider culture that emerged. In many respects, the parental campaign for rights and respect was personal but focused on public policy. Beginning in the 1950s, families helped to create a formidable coalition with attorneys, social workers, and the residents themselves that led to the closure of Pennhurst and similar state facilities.

The visual image of sturdy Jacobian buildings and manicured lawns, paired with the professional insistence that this was the best life they could give their child, might have persuaded parents that Pennhurst was a suitable setting. Desperation mixed with feelings of guilt influenced family decisions on placement. At least until the 1950s, when organizations like the National Association for Retarded Children (today known as the Arc of the United States) sought to inspect conditions, public access to Pennhurst and other institutions was usually denied. When rumors and more substantive evidence of mistreatment surfaced, parental hopes for their children (even adult children) eroded, replaced by a determination to take corrective measures.

Eleanor Elkin, a founding member of the Arc of Pennsylvania and later president of the Arc of the United States, is a case in point.[6] She and her husband Phil became aware of the plight of parents and families when in 1948 they became guardians of a two-month-old child whom they named Richard. None of the medical staff at the local hospital expected Richard to survive. He did, but it quickly became apparent that he had an intellectual disability. In spite of his delays, Richard brought immense joy to the entire family and they loved him unconditionally.

By the time Richard turned four, Elkin experienced firsthand the frustration, sorrow, and anguish that many parents felt from this era. The family never legally adopted Richard, because a local judge insisted that it would not be "fair" to his sister, Margo, and her future inheritances. Consequently, when Eleanor requested a preschool program with transportation to enhance Richard's learning abilities, the county officials said that they had a better idea: send Richard to the Judge School in the Poconos. Despite Eleanor's protests, they took Richard out of her loving arms and sent him to a segregated institution in northeast Pennsylvania. Eleanor's sister, who had recently lost a child due to a heart problem, sadly stated that "watching Richard being sent away was worse than having a baby die."

In a development that was representative of institutional responses to parents' inquiries, Eleanor was unable to visit Richard for almost six months. This estrangement was compounded by the outbreak of polio at Pennhurst. Eleanor sent Richard letters, toys, and candy with instructions to share them with the other children. She received a return letter shortly stating, "Do not send any more packages. If everyone did that, the staff would not get their work done." At home, Richard's absence affected Margo. She would sneak into her parents' bedroom late at night and quietly lay on the floor beside their bed, afraid that they might send her away, too.

When the Elkins finally received permission to visit Richard, they noticed his health had declined dramatically and his torso protruded from malnutrition and hunger. A former employee of the Judge School told them Richard lived off a diet of bread and molasses. Furious, the Elkins took action and tearfully went before a judge to plea for Richard's release. They finally succeeded in bringing Richard home. In 2008, after living a fulfilling life, Richard Elkin died of natural causes at the age of sixty while surrounded by a loving family.[7]

In the fall of 1950, forty-two parent representatives met in Minneapolis in the hope of joining forces to improve state centers for individuals with intellectual disabilities. As one parent-participant exclaimed: "Imagine it! Practically every parent there thought his group was the pioneer. Most of us were strangers to each other—suspicious of everyone's motives and jealous of their progress. . . . These parents, all strangers to each other, without money, precedent, or policy to follow, united with the purpose and "common goal—to help ALL 'retarded' children and their parents."[8]

These parent-advocates established the National Association of Parents and Friends of Mentally Retarded Children (later to become simply the National Association of Retarded Children [NARC]). The new organization's slogan proclaimed, "Retarded children CAN be helped"[9] Within fifteen years, NARC had more than 218,000 members in 1,700 chapters. Supported by the Kennedy administration and the President's Committee on Mental Retardation, advocates and their own expert advisors challenged medical authorities and policymakers who had instructed them to institutionalize and forget about their children. In existence since 1949, the Pennsylvania group affiliated with the national organization (ARC) in 1951.

"It began in 1949," Elkin explained of the Pennsylvania parent's organization, "when a mother put an ad in the Philadelphia newspaper asking for other mothers who might have children with intellectual disabilities who had been excluded from school. Mothers didn't know what to do with their children, and they were seeking help." Eight parents responded to this letter and after initially sharing their concerns around kitchen tables, they started holding regular meetings at the office of Yale and Juliet Nathanson in Philadelphia. Incorporated as a nonprofit organization on October 17, 1949, the all-volunteer Pennsylvania Association for Retarded and Handicapped Children (later known simply as PARC) targeted the right to public education and rehabilitative services as essential to the welfare of children with mental and physical disabilities, "regardless of race, creed, color or national origin." The charter also stressed the necessity of trained medical and behavioral specialists to work with children to reach their individual potentials.

A powerful philosophy supported Pennsylvania advocacy: (1) children with intellectual disabilities *could* be helped, (2) it was a public responsibility to provide such services, and (3) these services could be established through the organized activities of this parent group. On the eve of statewide organizations' affiliation with NARC in 1951, five counties in southeastern Pennsylvania united with the Pennsylvania

Association for Retarded and Handicapped Children and incorporated as the Pennsylvania Association for Retarded Children (PARC). Soon after, other organizations from across the Commonwealth joined the cause and pledged to work for a better life for *all* people with intellectual disabilities.

This flurry of parental and organizational advocacy was assisted by noted author Pearl Buck. According to Elkin, "Parents from all over southeastern Pennsylvania came to hear her [Buck] speak. They really got on fire with ideas of things that could be done. They went back and formed their own local chapters." Buck was the bestselling author of *The Good Earth* (1931), a Pulitzer Prize recipient in 1935, and the first American woman to win the Nobel Prize for literature. Buck's daughter, Carol, was diagnosed with an intellectual disability, later attributed to phenylketonuria (PKU). After years of searching for a cure and the fear that Carol's condition was indicative of failure, Pearl accepted her daughter's condition and continued to write while trying to find an appropriate residential placement for Carol. According to Elkin, "Pearl supported community residences, but also viewed institutionalization favorably." Despite Buck's generally positive attitude toward institutionalization, she struggled to find an institution to meet Carol's needs. Visits and interviews left "discouraging impressions . . . many schools were managed as warehouses, in which children were simply stored until they died."[10] She eventually chose the Vineland Training School in New Jersey due to its proximity to her home in Philadelphia.

Pearl Buck's personal experience led her to do what writers do—in 1950 she published a magazine piece in *Ladies' Home Journal* that became a book about Carol entitled *The Child Who Never Grew Up*.[11] Appearing at the dawn of the parental advocacy era, Buck's compelling personal account gave families hope, recognition, and the determination to move forward. By 1958, Pearl Buck's celebrity status had led to her appointment as chair of the Governor's Committee on Handicapped Children.

In a similar vein, actor Roy Rogers, the "King of the Cowboys," and his wife, Dale Evans, gained national recognition in their own advocacy efforts. In 1950, this movie and television superstar couple gave birth to a daughter named Robin. Even though Robin was born with Down syndrome, Roy and Dale did not shy away from public attention to their child and her needs. "In those days people saw an offspring as evidence of genetic weakness in the parents," Dale wrote.[12] She went on to say, using the terminology of the day, "Mongoloid children were usually hidden because society was not willing to accept them. . . . But God knew that if we would accept the challenge of caring for Robin, he could use us to witness of his love in new and exciting ways."

Dale and Roy were devastated when Robin died a day short of her second birthday due to complications with mumps. Roy later said, "The hardest thing I ever did was look at my daughter in that coffin . . . she looked like a small-size sleeping angel." Displaying their deep religious convictions, Dale wrote *Angel Unaware* in 1953, to share the belief that "Robin came from God—an angel—with all her handicaps and frailties to make us aware that his strength is found in weakness." She encouraged readers to "find transcendent meaning in mental retardation" while suggesting "all special children should be kept at home. Angels have a purpose that is lost in an institution."[13]

*Angel Unaware* became a national bestseller, going through thirty printings with all the royalties—over $20,000 in the first year alone—donated to the newly formed National Association for Retarded Children. With the funds, the parent advocacy group opened up offices in New York City.[14] To this day, royalties continue to flow into the Washington, D.C., office of the Arc of the United States. In the past half century, many prominent individuals have volunteered or made financial contributions to the Arc and its state chapters. Some have been parents of children with intellectual and developmental disabilities, and others simply people of goodwill who have been recruited to the advocacy cause. Well-known figures who have supported the Arc include Cliff Robertson, Tony Orlando, Frank Gifford, Barbara Walters, Carol Burnett, Barbara Streisand, Bill Cosby, Carol Channing, Michael Landon, and Geraldo Rivera, and members of the Kennedy and Shriver families, to name a few.

## The Pennsylvania Experience

In Pennsylvania prior to 1950, all children with IQ scores below fifty were excluded from the public school system and assigned instead to the Department of Public Welfare. Providing services to these children was one of the earliest activities for this new state association. At first, parents offered each other informal sitter services, but soon classes for the so-called "orthogenically backward," known as "Opportunity Classes," were established around the state. Eleanor remembers raising funds through bake sales to start nursery classes and schools in church basements and fought to secure programs for children who were labeled "uneducable." She recalled in 2010, "These mothers became volunteer teachers and even supplied the toys. The churches were very kind to let us have a place to do this. That led to parents getting a little bit brave and deciding, 'Gee, we could go to the school board. Why shouldn't they be doing some of this?'"

By 1954, legislation was approved permitting, but not mandating, local public school districts to provide classes and assist with the arrangements for those children with IQs under fifty. Elkin recalled, "The school boards, in some cases, listened to us and said 'Well, okay, we'll hire a teacher, but you have to supply all of the materials and fix up the room in the basement, supply the desks and you have to put a bathroom in, etc.' Well, we did that. People in the community helped and we were able to get a few classes going. With trained teachers, this really meant something to us. What we learned at this period of time would help us a great deal when we started the right to education [campaign]." Elkin continued: "Not only did we reach out to families who had their children at home, but also to families who had children in institutions. We couldn't get into the institutions, we were not welcome. We formed institution committees which later became residential committees. The committees were not welcomed by the administration because they considered them threatening. They were also worried about protecting the privacy of families and children."

Elkin and other leaders formed "Sunshine Committees" for the children at the Polk, Pennhurst, and Laurelton institutions. They sent cards, without names, for birthdays and at Christmas, and they left small gifts at the main office. Staff characterized the efforts of these volunteers as "outside interference" and discouraged them under the guise of privacy. PARC funded shows by traveling circuses and even swimming pools for the institutionalized children.

The repeal of Jim Crow racial segregation laws, beginning with the U.S. Supreme Court's landmark *Brown v. Board of Education* decision (1954), which invalidated "separate but equal" public education based on race, paved the way for a movement toward civil rights for persons with intellectual disabilities. A challenge based on the equal protection and due process clauses seemed to offer a means of attacking the legal segregation and the exclusion of children with disabilities from public schools (see chapter 6). However, it would be twenty years before the constitutional mandate of equal educational access would be addressed by the state and federal courts. Pennhurst figured prominently in that struggle.

Meanwhile, parents were gaining strength and learning the skills of leadership and advocacy. At times, the problems facing PARC volunteers seemed insurmountable, requiring a greater degree of organizational expertise. In order to meet the growing demands, standing committees were established in the areas of education, legislation, institutions, organizations, fundraising, public relations, and recreation. Advocates also worked toward funding for research and the publication of a newsletter.

By 1955, the Pennsylvania Association for Retarded Children (PARC) had grown to forty-one local chapters. Along with the nationwide organization (NARC), the Pennsylvania chapter made important strides in the field of intellectual disabilities. The multifaceted activities of PARC and its increasing volunteer base made it necessary to hire the first state executive director, Mr. Harry Blank.

In Pennsylvania in the mid-1950s, nine thousand children were living in state institutions, and another three thousand were on waiting lists for placement. Seventy applications for residential placement were being received each month. As previously noted, the Pennhurst population had peaked at an all-time high of 3,500. PARC had already developed a reputation of expertise in the field of education for children with intellectual disabilities. The association was able to pull in federal funding through the Rehabilitation Act of 1954, which assisted states in meeting the costs of research, demonstration projects, and training. This federal funding helped to gain state funding to begin the establishment of some chapter-operated sheltered employment. "Sheltered" in this context refers to employment settings intended to teach people with disabilities useful skills. Also, because of PARC's emerging credibility, volunteers began touring state institutions with government officials, which revealed severe overcrowding.[15] Reflecting back on this period, Eleanor Elkin recalled in 1976:

> When parents were finally able to go inside institutions, they didn't like what they saw. Something had to be done and the struggle for change began. It was not easy, especially for the parents who had placed their children there years ago. After all, they were told that putting their children away was the only thing to do and it's hard to reverse a decision that was very painfully made. . . . I visited Selinsgrove State School and Hospital, north of Harrisburg. It was not a very attractive building. But it was new and shiny. They had children, 2 and 3 years old, in cribs and playpens, but mostly in cribs. I asked, "Why are they in cribs?" "Well, if we don't keep them in cribs, they will get out and run around all over the place." Seemed to me, that's what children were supposed to do, so I didn't think too much of Selinsgrove.[16]

Her reaction was much the same at Pennhurst and other facilities:

> Some of Pennhurst's residents moved to White Haven State School [White Haven, in the mountains of northeastern Pennsylvania, was known as Pennhurst State School Annex #2, a subdivision of the Pennhurst State School and Hospital at Spring City, PA]. But that didn't work either, because they were still moving them into another institution, it was not a place in the community where they could live, play and go to school with other kids. We weren't helping the people that we were working so hard to help. We just couldn't do it that way, and we knew that we had to go a different route.[17]

Volunteers began demanding that institutions shift their emphasis from basic custodial care to rehabilitation and training. Parents who were unable to pay for their child's institutional care had government property liens placed on their own homes. PARC volunteers were successful in getting the Liens Bill passed to finally give these families protection and financial relief.

In 1957, an influenza epidemic struck and caused the death of many Pennhurst residents. At PARC's insistence, the Departments of Health and Welfare instituted an immunizations program for all residents. By 1960, additional grants for sheltered workshops (for employment) were awarded to local chapters of PARC. The movement was building momentum, but not fast enough. Many children and adults in the community were still without services, including public education, and the institutions were vastly overcrowded. Parents were desperate to work with government officials in a cooperative manner. Although they wanted so much more for all children, they feared losing the strides they had already made by pushing too hard.

Local PARC chapters continued to be busy in the 1960s, building and staffing schools, classes, daycare centers, vocational programs, and other services, and providing alternatives for families. Through PARC's efforts, the PKU newborn screening law was passed and the State's Office of Mental Retardation was established, finally separating its role from the Mental Health Office. State government funding flowed in for community residential living programs. Critics noted that the meager funds were inadequate to correct historic overcrowding and improve existing facilities and those under construction.

The 1966 publication of *Christmas in Purgatory*, a disturbing photo-essay on institutional life, upset readers. Authors Burton Blatt and Fred Kaplan visited five institutions and concluded, "There is a hell on earth, and in America there is a special inferno. We were visitors there during Christmas, 1965."[18] Their indictment of institutionalization went further, echoing Senator Robert Kennedy's assessment but with images to illustrate the point.

Three years later, in the summer of 1968, local news reporter Bill Baldini produced his five-part, groundbreaking exposé on Pennhurst

State School and Hospital. This was the first time that actual video footage focusing on neglect and overcrowding was shown to an American television audience. The local public was shocked by the accounts, and Baldini was unable to host the fifth day because of fatigue and complete loss of voice. The footage also stirred PARC families to a new level of advocacy.

By November, PARC received a $25,000 grant from the Kennedy Foundation to conduct thorough visits of all Commonwealth institutions. Dennis Haggerty, a parent-advocate and chair of the volunteer residential care committee, remembered that PARC advocates accompanied by members of the Jaycees "could not believe what they saw." After their site visits, Haggerty said, "Some of them vomited." PARC Executive Board member L. Stuart Brown characterized Pennhurst in particular as "a Dachau, without ovens." According to his account: "Large numbers of retarded persons have been herded together to live as animals in a barn, complete with stench. Many are forced into slave labor conditions; deprived of privacy, affection, morality; suffering the indignities of nakedness, beatings, sexual assaults and exposure. Some are doped out of reality with chemical restraints while others are physically deformed by the mechanical ones. Many are sitting aimlessly without motivations, incentives, hopes, or programs."[19]

To commemorate the sixtieth anniversary of Pennhurst's opening, on November 29, 1968, the PARC Youth Corps organized a pilgrimage to the site. Accompanied by parent-advocates, over one thousand youth from all over the Commonwealth carried lit "candles of hope" and marched on Pennhurst to express their concern. Led by their president, Annette Zelder, the youth advocates pledged their personal commitment to bringing the residents of Pennhurst from the darkness of institutional despair into the light of hope. After viewing *Suffer the Little Children*, they returned to their communities with petitions of concern. Two months later, advocates held an all-night vigil on the steps of the State Capitol in Harrisburg. They also presented petitions signed by over two hundred thousand Pennsylvanians calling for immediate official action to abolish inhumane conditions and provide adequate care for the residents at Pennhurst and other state facilities. As another sign of the burgeoning grassroots movement, more than seventy thousand volunteers between the ages of thirteen and twenty-five became involved in Youth NARC projects across America, with the stated purpose: "to serve as a friend of mentally retarded persons . . . to help the retarded learn to live in, work in, and attempt to better his world."[20]

## The Crusade for Change: 1968 to 1972

At a critical juncture in the emerging disability rights movement, a remarkable group of parent-advocates directed the Pennsylvania Arc. Jim Wilson, with a stable and even-keeled personality, was voted in as president of PARC in 1968. Patricia "Pat" Clapp, who was instrumental in coordinating the Youth PARC, became first vice president. L. Stuart Brown, who pulled no punches, was its third vice president. Attorney Dennis Haggerty, a clever strategist who later served on the President's Committee on Mental Retardation, was named chairman of the Residential Care Committee. Equally important, their group's good friend and mentor, Eleanor Elkin, was elected president of the national Arc.

Pat Clapp's son David had been diagnosed with Down syndrome. She reminisced about this period preceding groundbreaking court litigation over individual rights: "We knew that there had to be a change, change in leadership, in attitudes, and in the system. We also knew that we couldn't do it alone within PARC. We had to reach out to others." The Jaycees were particularly important allies, active in the greater Philadelphia and Pittsburgh areas. "The JCs were wonderful and I loved their slogan, 'We didn't know it couldn't be done, so we did it."[21]

Borrowing the Jaycee's slogan, President Eleanor Elkin challenged delegates at the 1968 national convention in Detroit to launch the "Crusade for Change." She asserted "a major campaign must be carried out to eliminate the dehumanizing conditions in institutions for the retarded." With over four thousand local clubs, the General Federation of Women's Clubs donated over $1 million and a million-plus hours of volunteer time, according to Clapp. "That was the 'Crusade' and Eleanor started the national revolution!"[22]

Clapp had special respect for Dennis Haggerty. “He did a lot of the planning strategy and PARC president Jim Wilson kept us on base so that we all stayed in line and we delivered. It was a great period of time. We decided that we had to work on changing attitudes. We certainly felt that people needed to know what was going on,” she told an interviewer.[23]

Eleanor Elkin and Pat Clapp together visited Polk State School and Hospital north of Pittsburgh, and what they observed exceeded their worst expectations. Children and adults were straitjacketed and manacled to benches to restrain their movements. Of one nine-year-old girl, staff said it was to prevent self-injurious behavior and to protect others. Clapp had a daughter the same age, and to “see a small child in such a condition was just terrible.” There was a five-foot-by-five-foot wooden cage, and its three-foot-high door was padlocked closed. Within sat an elderly woman clutching a baby doll in her arms, confined because she would not surrender the doll when so instructed by the staff. “And that was my feeling,” Clapp said, “man's inhumanity to man—how can you put people in cages like animals?”

Pat Clapp remembered on her visit, “The one that really got to me was going into the ward where there were wall to wall baby cribs, and the babies were laying there with no covers on the mattresses, crying. How in the world could they feed and love and care for those babies? And then it brought to mind our son, who was born in 1955. That's what they told us to do with David, they said, ‘Place him in an institution.’ So as I looked at those babies, I thought that could have been the life of our son, if we hadn't decided differently.”[24] (It is worth noting that thirty years later, in the spring 1999, five Polk physicians were indicted on charges ranging from malpractice to manslaughter in the death of several residents, and the entire nursing staff was brought before a local magistrate.[25])

The sad accounts of visits to Pennsylvania institutions were shared within PARC committees. Fearful of losing their own funding for community programs, some local chapters balked at more confrontational advocacy. However, at the Nineteenth Annual PARC Convention in Pittsburgh, in May 1969, President Jim Wilson confronted conditions head-on in an address entitled “High Time to Stop Hoping, Time to Act!" His call to action gained national exposure when reprinted in the PARC newsletter. "What should PARC's role be in the years ahead?" Wilson asked. "First, we should not reflect on the changes taking place around us. We should initiate change, act as an agent of change. . . . Very simply, we have a hunting license to innovate. It's up to us!"[26]

During the convention's business meeting, Dennis Haggerty showed graphic slides of a young man with severe disabilities, badly burned, in a morgue at Pennhurst. The photos were taken during an undercover investigation. The news of the death did not reach his mother until she attempted to visit him ten months later—on Thanksgiving Day. After waiting for three hours at Pennhurst's front desk, she was given the 'official' story that her son, John Stark Williams, died after slipping in the shower. Before she left, a boy ran out and told her, "Johnny died in a fire." This testimony catapulted PARC's board into action.[27]

Dennis Haggerty's photos from Pennhurst "did the final sell" to PARC leadership, but the debate was strong and bitter. Before the 1969 convention closed, a resolution written by Haggerty and the Residential Care Committee, along with five chapters in southeastern Pennsylvania, was brought back to the business session. Delegates voted to "authorize immediate retention of counsel by the Association for the filing of such legal action against the Department of Public Welfare as is necessary to either have it close Pennhurst or show just cause for its continuance." The resolution, which evolved into Pennsylvania's "Right to Education" case, passed unanimously.[28]

Dr. Gunnar Dybwad, beloved former executive director of NARC and professor of human development at Brandeis University, challenged the Pennsylvania chapter to frame disability issues as a civil rights cause, not merely a medical condition. Dybwad and his wife, Rosemary, were cofounders of Inclusion International, a highly respected global disability rights organization. In a now-famous speech to the Pennsylvania delegates, Dybwad asked about the conference theme, "Partners in Progress." "Let me ask you a very blunt question," he said. "What Progress? And Which Partners? For nineteen years you have tried to be nice. You've kept quiet too long." He ended his remarks with what would be a telling prediction: "You have adopted a resolution with which you finally take the first steps to assure for Pennsylvania's retarded citizens some rights in their own country. This resolution to retain counsel to determine what legal action you as an association can take against the Pennsylvania Department of Public Welfare to either close Pennhurst or justify its continuance is what you should do."[29]

Not everyone was comfortable with Dybwad's recommendation to sue the Commonwealth of Pennsylvania, what would become *PARC v. Commonwealth of Pennsylvania*. Among other concerns, there was great trepidation over what might replace Pennhurst and the other facilities. Peter Polloni, PARC's executive director, remembered, "Many were afraid and intimidated that change would be too difficult. People like Pat Clapp took a lot of abuse by bitter communications from some parents and certainly by the union people involved in the institutions." Where would the residents go? Several state leaders resigned from the organization. Parent-advocates like Polly Spare, a board member with two children at Pennhurst, later went on to create a new national organization, "The Voice of the Retarded," dedicated to keeping institutions as a viable option for parents.

Despite the resistance, in late 1969, Philadelphia civil rights attorney Thomas K. Gilhool (later Pennsylvania secretary of education) was retained to prepare a legal brief and sue the Commonwealth over conditions at Pennhurst. The Yale-educated attorney had a brother, David, who had lived in an institution since the age of ten. Mindful of the precedent established in the 1954 *Brown* decision, Gilhool recommended the PARC Board file a civil rights lawsuit to secure the residents' right to a public education. Dr. Dybwad convinced PARC that this strategy might be a way to eventually close all institutions by drying up the demand.

PARC's Executive Committee accepted the recommendation and authorized Gilhool to proceed. On Friday, May 5, 1972, a consent agreement was signed between PARC and the Commonwealth of Pennsylvania mandating that "retarded children must be afforded the free public education originally legislated in 1955."[30] PARC's Jim Wilson recalled, "Several years after the PARC settlement, Justice

Rehnquist of the U.S. Supreme Court said, 'the impetus for the Education for All Handicapped Children Act, now IDEA, came from the PARC litigation.'"[31]

The legal victory was a triumph for organizational advocacy in defense of the rights of citizens with intellectual and developmental disabilities. It also demonstrated the power of persistent parental and family engagement with critical issues of public policy. A subtle but significant shift in emphasis validated the experiences of individuals who lived in institutions and overcame the abuse and misfortune of being merely "put away." The examples set by Eleanor Elkin, Pat Clapp, future Pennsylvania first lady Ginny Thornburgh, to say nothing of the persuasive advocacy of Dennis Haggerty, Jim Wilson, and attorneys like Thomas Gilhool and David Ferleger, confronted social stigma and laid the foundations for a better life beyond Pennhurst and similar institutions. In time, residents themselves would speak out in a movement for self-advocacy that had its own profound impact on disability policy at the national and state level.

## Notes

1. "Living Peace in a Time of War: The Civilian Public Service Story," Mennonite Central Committee, http://civilianpublicservice.org; "List of CPS Camps," Swarthmore College Peace Collection, https://www.swarthmore.edu/library/peace/conscientiousobjection/CPScampsList.htm; Joseph Shapiro, "WWII Pacifists Exposed Mental Ward Horrors," *NPR*, December 30, 2009, http://www.npr.org/templates/story/story.php?storyId=122017757. For a general overview, see also Jeffery Kovacs, *Refusing War, Affirming Peace: A History of Civilian Public Service Camp #21 at Cascade Locks* (Eugene: Oregon State University Press, 2009).

2. Joseph Shapiro, "WWII Pacificists Exposed Mental Ward Horrors," https://www.npr.org/templates/story/story.php?storyId=122017757.

3. Steven J. Taylor, *Acts of Conscience: World War II, Mental Institutions, and Religious Objectors* (Syracuse: Syracuse University Press, 2009); James W. Trent, *Inventing the Feeble Mind: A History of Mental Retardation in the United States* (Los Angeles: University of California Press, 1994).

4. Taylor, *Acts of Conscience*, 266.

5. Joanne R. Pompano, *The Path to Opportunity: A Study of Disability Rights in Postwar America*, Yale-New Haven Teachers Insitute (curriculum unit 06.03.07), http://teachersinstitute.yale.edu/curriculum/units/2006/3/06.03.07.x.html.

6. Eleanor Elkin sat for an extended interview with Lisa Sonneborn and the Temple University "Visionary Voices" project, n.d., http://www.temple.edu/instituteondisabilities/voices/detailVideo.html?media=005-01; National Association for Retarded Children, *Annual Conference: Crusade for Change* (1968), n.p.; Eleanor Elkin, interviews by Janet Albert-Herman, April, 2011.

7. Eleanor Elkin, remarks delivered at 2011 historical marker dedication ceremony, Spring City, April 2011.

8. "A History of the National Association for Retarded Children, Inc.," (web page discontinued).

9. President's Committee on Mental Retardation, *Mental Retardation Past and Present*, MR 77 (Washington, D.C.: Government Printing Office, 1977), 40.

10. Peter Conn, *Pearl S. Buck: A Cultural Biography* (New York: Cambridge University Press, 1998), 111.

11. Pearl Buck, *The Child Who Never Grew Up* (New York: John Day, 1950). The story originally was published in magazine syndication.

12. Anne Adams, "Dale Evans—Entertainer/Mother/Writer," History's Women, Amazing Moms, http://www.historyswomen.com/amazingmoms/DaleEvans.html.

13. Chris Enss and Howard Kazanijan, *The Cowboy and the Señorita: A Biography of Roy and Dale Evans* (Guildford, Conn.: TwoDot Press, 2005), 128, 236.

14. Gunnar Dybwad, "From Feebleminded to Self-Advocacy: A Half-Century of Growth and Self-Fulfillment," *Proceedings of the Annual Meeting of the American Association on Mental Retardation* (1994).

15. President's Committee on Mental Retardation, *Mental Retardation Past and Present*; Linda H. Drummond, ed., *ARC Pennsylvania: Historical Perspective Overview 1949 to 1990* (Harrisburg: ARC, 1990), 4–6.

16. Eleanor Elkin, interviews by Janet Albert-Herman, April, 2011.

17. Eleanor Elkin, remarks delivered at Pennhurst Historical Marker Dedication, April 10, 2010, Spring City, Pennsylvania.

18. Burton Blatt and Fred Kaplan, *Christmas in Purgatory: A Photographic Essay on Mental Retardation* (1965; Syracuse, N.Y.: Human Policy Press, 1974).

19. Leopold Lippman and I. Ignacy Goldberg, *Right to Education: Anatomy of the Pennsylvania Case and Its Implications* (New York: Teachers College Press, 1973), 17.

20. Drummond, *ARC Pennsylvania*, 5.

21. Clapp personal notes, in possession of Janet Albert-Herman; NARC, "Crusade for Change," in *Proceedings of Nineteenth Annual Meeting* (Detroit, 1968).

22. Ibid.

23. Clapp, interview with Janet Albert-Herman, n.d.

24. Clapp personal notes in possession of Janet Albert-Herman.

25. "State Charges Polk Doctors," *Pittsburgh Post-Gazette*, February 27, 1999, 1.

26. James Wilson, "High Time to Stop Hoping, Time to Act," *Pennsylvania Message* (1969): n.p.

27. Fred Pelka, *What We Have Done: An Oral History of the Disability Rights Movement* (Amherst: University of Massachusetts Press, 2012).

28. Ibid.

29. Remarks delivered at the 1969 annual convention and summarized in *Pennsylvania Message* (1969); copy in personal possession of the authors.

30. PARC Consent Decree 1972, available at http://thearcpa.org/resources/historical docs.html.

31. Jim Wilson, interview with Lisa Sonneborn for "Visionary Voices," December 16, 2011; https://disabilities.temple.edu/voices/detailVideo.html?media=018-01.

CHAPTER 6

# From PARC to Pennhurst

## *The Legal Argument for Equality*

JUDITH A. GRAN

The Pennsylvania Association for Retarded Children's (PARC's) decision to hire an attorney to advise them on the matter of institutonal abuse turned out to be world changing for the lives of the people at Pennhurst, and for their families. It also transformed how the law considered and respected citizens with disabilities. What happened in the courts that remedied the horrible problems at Pennhurst? Moreover, how did the legal work surrounding Pennhurst fundamentally improve the national legal approach to disability in the decades that followed? This chapter tells the legal story of lasting victories, including the background upon which the victories were founded.

### The Right to Education Based on Equal Protection of the Law

In the wake of the exposé by Bill Baldini of conditions at Pennhurst in 1968, the Pennsylvania Association for Retarded Children, or PARC, hired an attorney, Thomas K. Gilhool of Philadelphia, to analyze the various legal options and make a recommendation to the PARC board. Gilhool had extensive experience in civil rights litigation, including cases brought to enforce the Equal Protection Clause of the Fourteenth Amendment. He had recently argued a seminal Equal Protection case, *Shapiro v. Thompson*, before the Supreme Court.[1] Gilhool suggested that the most effective approach to challenging Pennhurst would be to stop children from being sent there—to "close the front door."[2]

In those days, most people being admitted to Pennhurst were children—and most of them were around the age of adolescence. Why children? Because children with any disabilities, particularly significant ones, were not welcome in public schools. It is hard to believe, but in those days children were sorted into groups labeled:

"Educable"—some hope for learning minor academics
"Trainable"—no hope for academic benefit whatsoever, but possibly able to be trained to take care of daily needs or perform routine functions
"Custodial"—no capacity for learning of any kind, hence to be relegated to custodial care aimed at life support, physical health, freedom from abuse and pain

Children in any of those three categories could be excluded from our public schools—educable the least, trainable perhaps half, and custodial nearly 100 percent.

Because so many children were kept out of public school, families of children with any kind of special needs struggled. Where should their children go every day? There was literally nothing in American communities. Someone in the family had to stay home every day, all day with the child. As young children became teenagers, the problems of such a family life multiplied. Developmental delays and behavioral challenges, to say nothing of the financial expense for therapeutic interventions, were among the issues that intensified a family's sense of social isolation. Whenever such a family approached a social agency for advice or help, the answer was quite consistent: the ONLY option offered by society was the nearest institution, in this case, Pennhurst. That is why most of the admissions to Pennhurst (and to every other institution in America) during this time were adolescents. It bears repeating that this difficult situation existed only because children with significant disabilities were not permitted to attend public school.

Perceiving this was part of the brilliance of the approach offered to PARC by attorney Gilhool. Thus the first step in any challenge to the existence of Pennhurst was to challenge the exclusion of children with intellectual disabilities from school.

Gilhool recommended that PARC file a lawsuit challenging the interpretation of state laws established in the late 1940s, which allowed school districts to exclude children with intellectual disabilities from school.[3] He likened these sections of the Pennsylvania School Code to the *de jure* segregation of African American children. Their exclusion from the public schools attended by other children was challenged successfully by the NAACP Legal Defense Fund in the systematically planned and executed series of lawsuits that culminated in *Brown v. Board of Education*.[4] In *Brown*, the Supreme Court held that providing separate schools for children of different races violated the Equal Protection Clause and ordered the regime of school segregation dismantled "with all deliberate speed."

The Court's application of the Equal Protection Clause in *Brown* did not depend on the abstract right to education, but rather the principle that once a state decides to educate the children within its borders, it must do so on an equal basis.[5] Significantly, the Court held that separate educational facilities were unequal even if the separate schools were comparable in physical facilities and other "tangible" measures: "Separate educational facilities are inherently unequal. Therefore, we hold that the plaintiffs and others similarly situated for whom the actions have been brought are, by reason of the segregation complained of, deprived of the equal protection of the laws guaranteed by the Fourteenth Amendment."[6]

Although *Brown* did not provide a solid basis for asserting a "right to treatment" for residents of Pennhurst, let alone a right to habilitation in the community, the PARC leadership understood from Gilhool's analysis that the most promising way to begin solving the problem of Pennhurst was to obtain the right to a public education for all children with intellectual disabilities. With these protections, families would not need to send children to institutions. PARC decided to file a lawsuit in federal court based on the Equal Protection Clause to obtain the right to the free, appropriate public education enjoyed by every other child in Pennsylvania. The action was filed in 1971.

In its decision, the three-judge district court in *PARC v. Commonwealth* adopted Gilhool's analysis that *de jure* exclusion of children with intellectual disabilities from public school violated the Equal Protection Clause. That decision and the settlement based on it became known in Pennsylvania, and later the nation, as the "Right to Education."

This legal victory spread rapidly. Families in every state were facing the same dilemma. The victory in Pennsylvania inspired other states. Lawsuits and policy changes swept the country. States began to recognize that all children belong to families and communities, and need not be "sent away." Once the snowballing of states' recognition of children's rights became irresistible, Congress acted. In 1975, Congress passed the "Education of All Handicapped Children Act"—and many years later in 1990, the name was changed to what we now know as IDEA, or the Individuals with Disabilities Education Act.

This is a wonderfully informative story, because today very few of us know that a lawsuit about horrendous institutional conditions brought about the realization that all of our nation's children should be included in schools—no matter what their origin, ethnicity, or disability status. It all began at Pennhurst.

It is useful to explain some of the history that led up to the PARC victory. That explanation makes it easier to understand how the next legal battle was chosen, and how it was won. The next legal battle was about actually closing Pennhurst, a case that began in 1974 and became known as *Halderman v. Pennhurst.*

The revolution in services for the residents of Pennhurst was preceded by a revolution in legal thought about the rights of persons with disabilities. Before the early 1970s, the federal courts—historically, the guardians of civil rights—had struggled to address abuse, lack of services, and horrific institutional conditions within the framework of the Constitution. The legal theories the courts employed were grounded in the due process clause of the Fourteenth Amendment, and they were characterized by a view of persons with disabilities as passive recipients of care and treatment. In contrast, the district court's approach in *Halderman v. Pennhurst* was grounded in the Equal Protection Clause and was characterized by a view of persons with disabilities as active citizens and persons who are created equal with their fellow citizens without disabilities.

The legal revolution that *Halderman v. Pennhurst* represented began in *PARC v. Commonwealth*. The fundamental Constitutional guarantee of equality lies at the heart of the consent decree that resolved that case.[7] *PARC* affirmed that all children, including those whose disabilities are most severe, are created equal.

The plaintiffs in *PARC* had asserted that the exclusion of children with intellectual disabilities from school violated the Equal Protection Clause. In approving the consent decree, the court held that the plaintiffs had stated a colorable claim for violation of the Equal Protection Clause and that the exclusion of students with intellectual disabilities from public school lacked any rational basis in fact.[8] The court found that these children had been excluded, not because they were "uneducable and untrainable," but because of the stigma attached to the label of "mental retardation," stigma with its roots in the eugenics movement[9] that began in the second decade of the twentieth century.[10] The provisions in the *PARC* decision were soon codified in federal legislation. The Education of All Handicapped Children Act,[11] now known as the Individuals with Disabilities Education Act (IDEA),[12] was enacted under Congress's power to enforce the Fourteenth Amendment's Equal Protection Clause.[13] In enacting the statute, Congress declared that its intent was to "assist State and local efforts to provide programs to meet the educational needs of handicapped children in order to assure equal protection of the law.[14]

In turn, the Equal Protection Clause is rooted in the fundamental American belief, first expressed in the Declaration of Independence, that all persons are created equal. In 1857, Abraham Lincoln declared in his speech on the Dred Scott decision, that the inclusion of this statement in the Declaration was forward looking. "They meant simply to declare the *right*, so that the *enforcement* of it might follow as fast as circumstances should permit. They meant to set up a standard maxim for free society, which should be familiar to all, and revered by all; constantly looked to, constantly labored for, and even though never perfectly attained, constantly approximated, and thereby constantly spreading and deepening its influence, and augmenting the happiness and value of life to all people of all colors everywhere."[15]

The liberation of citizens with disabilities from institutional confinement is part of the "constantly spreading and deepening" effect of the declaration of equality in our founding document. The knowledge that people with the most significant disabilities can live in and contribute to their communities as productive citizens means that they cannot be removed from their communities merely because of their differences or because they need support. That acknowledgment is the fundamental principle underlying two other Equal Protection statutes, Section 504 of the Rehabilitation Act of 1973,[16] which the district court applied in *Pennhurst*, and the Americans with Disabilities Act,[17] which was enacted after Pennhurst closed but defined civil rights protections for individuals with disabilities.

## The "Right to Treatment" and Other Legal Theories That Predated *PARC*

To appreciate how revolutionary the argument for equality that animated both *PARC* and *Pennhurst* was, it is helpful to look at the legal theories that courts and advocates employed in the litigation of the 1960s and 1970s that worked toward relief for the disabled living apart from society in institutions. Dominant early legal theories used in these cases included doctrines (1) based on the right to liberty, (2) based on the right to treatment or habilitation, and (3) based on the right to be free from harm or punishment. These doctrines appealed to lawyers who struggled to change the situation of people who were warehoused in large custodial institutions with little hope of release or living a normal life. However, each of these was problematic as a source of rights for institutionalized persons with disabilities. Even as they were embraced by some courts as a ground for holding the state liable for conditions in state institutions, they were rejected by others, including the United States Supreme Court. Critically, they provided little support for community placement as a remedy for institutional confinement, one of the primary causes in the advocacy movement. By the time *Halderman v. Pennhurst* had wended its way to the Supreme Court and back, these doctrines had run out of steam. First expressed in *PARC*, applied in *Pennhurst*, and finally codified in statutory form in Section 504 of the Rehabilitation Act and the Americans with Disabilities Act, the principle of equality has provided more solid ground for the dissolution of institutions and protection of community-based living alternatives.

## The Right to Liberty

Before *PARC v. Commonwealth*, most of the legal cases were built on the recognition that institutionalization is "a massive curtailment of liberty,"[18] and that the fundamental right to liberty under the due process clause forbids unjustified deprivation of that right. If liberty is deprived at the hands of the state, it must be justified by a permissible and legitimate state interest, which the state must establish in an appropriate proceeding.[19] Some of these early cases drew on a First Amendment case, *Shelton v. Tucker* (1960),[20] which held that a government aim, even a legitimate one, "cannot be pursued by means that broadly stifle fundamental personal liberties when the end can be more narrowly achieved. The breadth of legislative abridgment must be viewed in the light of less drastic means for achieving the same basic purpose."[21]

This doctrine interpreting the First Amendment right to freedom of expression became familiar in the institutional context as the doctrine that services should be provided in the "least restrictive environment." As the court pointed out in *Gary W. v. Louisiana* (1976), the term is "more a slogan than a constitutional doctrine."[22] In terms of human services, it was also extremely misleading. Over the years, this doctrine has had the unfortunate effect of justifying a "continuum" of services approach, in which services recipients are placed in various types of living arrangements (e.g., state institution, private congregate facility, group home, semi-independent living arrangement, one's own home) according to the intensity of their need for services. It is now understood that people with disabilities can receive services of almost any level of intensity in their own homes or other small homes in ordinary neighborhoods, and that indeed, people with the most complex disabilities have the greatest need for personalized services in small homes.

Cases invoking the right to liberty relied on the Fifth- and Fourteenth-Amendment guarantee that liberty cannot be denied without due process of law. Typically, the cases focused on procedural due process in the act of commitment. For example, in *Saville v. Treadway* (1974),[23] in which a young woman with disabilities successfully challenged the state's process for placing people with disabilities at Clover Bottom Hospital and School at the request of their parents and guardians, "without restriction," the Court held that "where individual liberty is at stake to the extent it is in the instant case, it is absolutely essential that such confinement be preceded by adequate procedural safeguards. Given the possible conflicts of interest between a mentally retarded child and even a parent, it seems obvious that the 'voluntary' commitment procedures [of state law] fall far short of those required by due process."

Similarly, in *Parham v. J. R.* (1979),[24] the U.S. Supreme Court recognized that "parents cannot always have absolute and unreviewable discretion to decide whether to have a child institutionalized." However, because this doctrine's primary remedy is the amendment of state commitment laws, it is not particularly helpful to institutionalized people with disabilities. Heightened procedural protections are unlikely to prevent the commitment of those with significant intellectual disabilities.

Other cases invoking the right to liberty relied on substantive due process. The Supreme Court's decisions in *Jackson v. Indiana* (1972),[25] and *O'Connor v. Donaldson* (1975)[26] were seminal decisions of the pre-*Pennhurst* era. In *Jackson*, the United States Supreme Court held that the nature and duration of involuntary confinement must bear some reasonable relationship to the rationale for commitment. *Jackson* challenged the constitutionality of a state commitment law that allowed the commitment of a Deaf man until he became competent to stand trial. Since he was unlikely ever to become competent, the Court held his indefinite commitment was improper. In *Donaldson*, which challenged an indefinite involuntary commitment to a mental hospital, the Supreme Court held that "a State cannot constitutionally confine . . . a nondangerous individual who is capable of surviving safely in freedom by himself or with the help of willing and responsible family members or friends." Similarly, the Court held that "mere public intolerance or animosity cannot constitutionally justify the deprivation of a person's physical liberty."

Although *Jackson* and *Donaldson* rested on a relatively firm constitutional foundation, the application of the doctrines announced in those cases to institutionalized persons with significant intellectual disabilities has been criticized by the courts. In *Garrity v. Gallen* (1981),[27] the district court noted that "unlike the [230] plaintiff in *O'Connor v. Donaldson*, . . . plaintiffs herein reside at [Laconia State School] because their family or friends are either unable or unwilling to care for them and because if left to the "hazards of freedom," they are "dangerous to (themselves)."[28] The district court accepted that "the state's willingness to provide the residents with such necessities as food, clothing, shelter, medical care, and supervision, for which the residents have no other source, forms an adequate basis for some state-imposed restrictions on their liberty."[29] In *Rogers v. Okin* (1980), the Court of Appeals held that caring for persons who need supervision is a proper reason for institutional confinement.

## The Right to Treatment or Habilitation

Throughout the 1960s and 1970s, the courts recognized that state institutions whose ostensible purpose was treatment, habilitation, or training offered little more than warehousing. By far the most popular legal doctrine of this period was the idea that in giving up one's liberty to the state, a person acquired a right to services. The term "right to treatment" was coined by Morton Birnbaum in his controversial 1960 article, "The Right to Treatment" (1960),[30] a work the *Pennhurst* court later called "seminal." Dr. Birnbaum proposed a "quid pro quo" theory as the foundation of a right to treatment. According to this concept, persons who are involuntarily confined because they need care and treatment trade their liberty for the services they need. Dr. Birnbaum advocated that the courts enforce the right to treatment "as necessary and overdue development of our present concept of due process of law."[31]

The first case declaring the existence of an enforceable right to treatment was *Rouse v. Cameron* (1966),[32] which applied Dr. Birnbaum's theory to a person seeking relief from involuntary commitment to an institution following his acquittal by reason of insanity. The court stated that since the purpose of involuntary hospitalization is treatment and not punishment, "involuntary confinement without treatment is 'shocking.'" The District of Columbia commitment statute under which the plaintiff was institutionalized required treatment for criminal defendants acquitted by reason of insanity, but even if it did not, the Court declared, the statute might violate the due process, equal protection, and cruel and unusual punishment clauses of the Constitution. The court found that the plaintiff was entitled to a hearing to determine whether he was receiving adequate treatment, and, if not, whether there was an overwhelmingly compelling reason for the failure to provide adequate treatment.

Subsequent cases applied the doctrine of a "right to treatment" to people with intellectual disabilities, holding that institutionalization created an enforceable "right to habilitation." In *Wyatt v. Aderholt* (1974),[33] the Court of Appeals held that failure to provide habilitation to persons with intellectual disabilities violates the due process clause. Similarly, in *Gary W. v. Louisiana* (1976), the district court held that involuntarily committed children with intellectual disabilities have a constitutional right to "a program of treatment that affords the individual a reasonable chance to acquire and maintain those life skills that enable him to cope as effectively as his own capacities permit with the demands of his own person and of his environment and to raise the level of his physical, mental and social efficiency."[34]

Courts derived the "right to treatment" from states' failure to provide the basic safeguards that criminal defendants must receive as a condition of incarceration: (1) strict procedural protections, (2) commitment of an offense for which punishment is appropriate, and (3) a limited duration of confinement.[35] According to the reasoning supporting the doctrine, treatment or habilitation is a compensation for the denial of any one of the basic safeguards.

The logic of this "quid pro quo" theory as a ground for enforcing the rights of institutionalized persons with intellectual disabilities is also problematic. The theory was developed to address the rights of persons with mental illness who were acquitted by reason of insanity and kept beyond the maximum possible sentence. In 1973, the court in *New York State Assoc. for Retarded Children, Inc. v. Rockefeller*[36] concluded that the quid pro quo theory that requires the state to "treat or release" could not easily be applied to institutionalized persons with intellectual disabilities, where release was not a realistic alternative. Requiring habilitation simply because those persons were in state custody would, in effect, impose a constitutional duty upon the state to provide services to its citizens, even if the Supreme Court held it was not required.[37]

This doctrine raised a number of challenges. If habilitation is offered as a trade-off for the denial of the basic procedural safeguards, it would follow that those procedural safeguards are not necessary to be provided, a proposition that the U.S. Supreme Court has rejected.[38] Conversely, if strict procedural safeguards are accorded before commitment, it would follow that habilitation need not be provided.[39] Further, the doctrine ignores the fact that the state may have reasons other than treatment or habilitation for confining some persons with disabilities, such as protection from harm or provision of custodial care,[40] where the court concluded that when the state commits an individual to an institution[41] solely to protect that person from harm, she or he is not entitled to treatment. At most, she would be entitled to protection from harming or injuring herself. Similarly, when a state in the exercise of its police power confines a person to an institution because he is dangerous to others, due process does not require that the state provide treatment.

The "quid pro quo" theory has been likened to the law of eminent domain, according to which the state may confiscate private property if it provides compensation in return.[42] The idea that the state may take away a person's liberty if it provides compensation in the form of treatment is a step that goes far beyond the principles of eminent domain and cannot be justified by any constitutional principle.

Another problem "right to treatment" theories faced was the discernment of an appropriate standard for judging the adequacy of the treatment available to people committed to insitutions involuntarily. Dr. Birnbaum himself emphasized that courts should not make judgments about the substantive adequacy of the treatment provided to an institutionalized individual, but he suggested that courts rely instead on formal standards, such as the number of staff, the adequacy of the physical facilities, and the frequency of professional consultations. Dr. Birnbaum considered that requiring more than the minimum formal standards of professional or accrediting organizations would open a Pandora's box.[43]

The most fundamental flaw of the "right to treatment" theories was their failure to challenge the institutional model. They failed to take into account the growing professional knowledge that people with significant intellectual disabilities could not be habilitated in large custodial institutions. The District Court in *Halderman v. Pennhurst* adopted the "right to treatment" theory, but with a significant variation. It held that "when a state involuntarily commits retarded persons, it must provide them with such habilitation as will afford them a reasonable opportunity to acquire and maintain those life skills necessary to cope as effectively as their capacities permit."[44] But it went on to find, based on the record made at trial, that adequate habilitation could not be provided in an institution such as Pennhurst: "As the Court has heretofore found, Pennhurst does not provide an atmosphere conducive to normalization which is so vital to the retarded if they are to be given the opportunity to acquire, maintain and improve their life skills. Pennhurst provides confinement and isolation, the antithesis of habilitation."[45]

## Institutionalization as Cruel and Unusual Punishment

A variation of right-to-treatment theories derived the right not from the individual liberties surrendered at commitment but from the Eighth- and Fourteenth-Amendment right to be free from cruel and unusual punishment. This theory was based on the Supreme Court's 1962 decision in *Robinson v. California*,[46] in which the Court struck down a state law allowing incarceration solely on the basis of an individual's status, in that case narcotics addiction, holding that punishment for one's status or condition constitutes cruel and unusual punishment.

The district court in *Welsch v. Likins* (1974),[47] applied *Robinson* to derive a right to treatment for people with intellectual disabilities who had been committed to a state institution, and held that since they had not been found guilty of a criminal offense, confining them without treatment violated the cruel and unusual punishment and due process clauses of the Constitution. Although the Court in *Robinson* had focused upon the status of narcotics addiction as a *criminal* offense,[48] rather than a basis for civil commitment, the court in *Welsch* held that the plaintiffs' "detention for mere illness—without a curative program" would constitute punishment for "status."[49]

The district court in *New York State Association for Retarded Children, Inc. v. Rockefeller* (1973)[50] rejected the concept of a right to treatment and declined to hold that those institutionalized because they needed care and supervision were entitled to treatment or habilitation. However, the court found that the residents of Willowbrook, who were "confined behind locked gates" and "held without the possibility of a meaningful waiver of their right to freedom," were entitled to at least the same living conditions as prisoners. The court found it unnecessary to decide whether this right was based on the Eighth Amendment, the Due Process Clause or the Equal Protection Clause, although it suggested that it might constitute an "irrational discrimination" between prisoners and innocent persons with disabilities to deny them rights that prisoners are accorded under the Eighth Amendment (conditions that protect from physical harm or deterioration).[51] Prefiguring Judge Broderick's opinion in *Halderman v. Pennhurst*, the court found that the state did have an obligation not to worsen an individual's condition.[52]

The theory of the Eighth Amendment as a source of rights for institutionalized persons with disabilities ran aground when the Supreme Court suggested, in *Ingraham v. Wright* (1977),[53] that the Eighth Amendment applies only to criminal punishment, although the Court noted that it was not deciding "whether or under what circumstances persons involuntarily confined in mental or juvenile institutions can claim the protection of the Eighth Amendment."[54] Since the Eighth Amendment doctrine rests on the assumption that commitment constitutes punishment, it is also difficult to reconcile with the language in *Robinson v. California*, which suggests that it would be acceptable for a state to determine that "the general health and welfare" required "compulsory treatment . . . confinement, or sequestration" for the mentally ill or other "victims . . . of other human afflictions."

## Judge Broderick Holds That Confinement Was Separate and Not Equal

After resolving *PARC v. Commonwealth*, PARC made plans for a follow-up suit on behalf of institutional residents and chose Pennhurst State School and Hospital as the target of the proposed litigation. Because its goal was to create opportunities for community living for institutional residents, *PARC* decided to await the construction of the Pennsylvania Mental Health / Mental Retardation Act of 1966 in a case in the Court of Common Pleas of Allegheny County during 1974.[55] This case centered on whether the placement of Joyce Z. in a state institution in western Pennsylvania was appropriate. Ginny Thornburgh's testimony on behalf of Joyce Z. convinced the court that conditions at the state institution would be harmful and that she could be served more appropriately in the community.

Meanwhile, *Halderman v. Pennhurst* was filed later that year by David Ferleger, a Philadelphia attorney with great expertise in disability rights, on behalf of Pennhurst residents. Ferleger, the son of two Holocaust survivors, had a deep and abiding interest in protecting people with disabilities from the harm that ensues when society's institutions fail to recognize their humanity. In 1975, PARC intervened as a plaintiff in the case; the United States, represented by lawyers from the Civil Rights Division of the United States Department of Justice, also became a plaintiff party. The case was filed as an action seeking damages for the egregious harm and abuse experienced by Pennhurst residents, with PARC seeking community placement. The representatives of all three sets of plaintiffs quickly came to consensus that the goal of the litigation should be the creation of a network of Community Living Arrangements (CLAs) where all residents of Pennhurst could receive services in typical homes, communities, and neighborhoods. In 1976, PARC attorney Tom Gilhool and David Ferleger jointly drafted and filed an amended complaint that reflected this goal.

By the time *Halderman v. Pennhurst* went to trial, legal scholars had already analyzed the implications of *PARC* for confinement of persons with intellectual disabilities in segregated institutions. Professor Robert Burt, asserted that the "*PARC* theory can and should mean that any state program that segregates mentally retarded citizens as such from others is highly suspect and that courts will require states to treat mentally retarded persons indistinguishably from others, except in ways that are both very limited and very clearly beneficial to the individual. . . . It is central to the inquiry into whether separate treatment for the mentally retarded person is not inherently unequal just as racially segregated education was found inherently unequal in *Brown v. Board of Education*."[56]

The plaintiffs' attorneys in *Pennhurst*, led by Tom Gilhool, made this argument to the district court, and the court adopted it, citing Professor Burt's article approvingly. In his initial opinion following the trial, Judge Raymond J. Broderick held that segregation at Pennhurst violated the Equal Protection Clause because it was both separate and unequal: "In this record, the evidence has been 'fully marshaled' and we find that the confinement and isolation of the retarded in the institution called Pennhurst is segregation in a facility that clearly is separate and *not* equal. . . . Thus, on the basis of this record we find that the retarded at Pennhurst have been and presently are being denied their Equal Protection Rights as guaranteed by the *Fourteenth Amendment to the Constitution*."

Judge Broderick accepted this case as a "class action," meaning that it would apply not just to the handful of complainants, but to other people in similar situations. Far broader in scope, individuals in this defined class were from then on referred to as "Pennhurst Class Members." Then he also held that segregation of class members at Pennhurst violated Section 504 of the Rehabilitation Act of 1973,[57] which prohibits discrimination in the following terms: "No otherwise qualified handicapped individual in the United States, as defined in section 706(6) of this title, shall, solely by reason of his handicap, be excluded from the participation in, be denied the benefits of, or be subjected to discrimination under any program or activity receiving Federal financial assistance." He held that in enacting

Section 504, "Congress has in effect codified the constitutional right to equal protection." He noted that the sponsors of Section 504 were particularly concerned about institutional segregation as a form of discrimination, citing the statement of Senator Hubert Humphrey, the bill's primary sponsor in the Senate, when he introduced the bill:

> The time has come when we can no longer tolerate the invisibility of the handicapped in America. . . . I am calling for public attention to . . . the Nation's institutionalized mentally retarded, who live in public and private residential facilities which are more than 50 years old, functionally inadequate, and designed simply to isolate these persons from society. . . . These people have the right to live, to work to the best of their ability—to know the dignity to which every human being is entitled. But too often we keep children, whom we regard as "different" or a "disturbing influence" out of our schools and community activities altogether. . . . Where is the cost-effectiveness in consigning them to . . . "terminal" care in an institution?[58]

Based on the finding that Section 504 codifies the rights recognized in the Equal Protection Clause and that the statute imposes affirmative obligations on state and local governmental officials, the court held that "under Section 504 unnecessarily separate and minimally inadequate services are discriminatory and unlawful."[59]

Judge Broderick's holdings that confinement of class members at Pennhurst violated the Equal Protection Clause and Section 504 of the Rehabilitation Act were never reversed or vacated, despite appeals in various courts, including the Supreme Court. Throughout those appeals, the District Court's orders remained in effect and implementation proceeded until the case was settled in 1984.

*Pennhurst* was followed by a wave of successful cases seeking community placement in states ranging from New Hampshire, Vermont, Rhode Island, Maine, Connecticut, North Carolina, and Michigan, to North Dakota, Texas, Oklahoma, and New Mexico, as well as the District of Columbia. Most of these cases resulted in settlement, and some resulted in favorable decisions for institutional residents under Section 504 (courts are advised not to decide cases on Constitutional grounds if the same result can be obtained under a statute).[60]

By highlighting the harms of institutionalization and separation from society, *Pennhurst* paved the way for passage of the Americans with Disabilities Act in 1990.[61] The ADA squarely defined segregation as a form of discrimination, stating in its Findings and Purpose: "The Congress finds that historically, society has tended to isolate and segregate individuals with disabilities, and, despite some improvements, such forms of discrimination against individuals with disabilities continue to be serious and pervasive social problems."[62] The ADA regulations forbid state and local governments to "provide different or separate aids, benefits, or services to individuals with disabilities or to any class of individuals with disabilities than is provided to others unless such action is necessary to provide qualified individuals with disabilities with aids, benefits, or services that are as effective as those provided to others."[63]

In its landmark decision in *Olmstead v. L. C.* (1999),[64] the U.S. Supreme Court applied the ADA regulation prohibiting unnecessary segregation to a case in which two women who had been confined in an institution in Georgia went to court to establish their right to receive services in the community. The plaintiffs won and the justices held that institutional segregation is an act of discrimination and a clear violation of the ADA's integration mandate: "Unjustified isolation . . . is properly regarded as discrimination based on disability."[65] The logical consequence, the Court held, is that "proscription of discrimination may require placement of persons with mental disabilities in community settings rather than institutions."[66] Those circumstances exist, the Court held, when the institutionalized person is "qualified" to live in a community setting, "with or without reasonable modifications" to the government entity's "rules, policies, or practices."[67]

The complete story of *Pennhurst*'s legacy in institutional litigation and its continuing impact on the courts in a new wave of post-*Olmstead* cases is long and will need to be told elsewhere. Suffice it to say that when we study and celebrate how the right to live in the community and to be free from institutional confinement became established, all roads lead back to *Pennhurst*—and *PARC*. It was in these cases that the courts recognized most powerfully that people with disabilities are not passive recipients of care and treatment but rather are created equal with their fellow citizens in every important respect.

## Notes

1. 394 U.S. 618 (U.S. 1969).

2. In a memorandum to PARC on possible litigation strategies, Gilhool identified five potential causes of action: (1) grievances of individual residents, (2) misdirection of the state's present capital expenditure plan, (3) involuntary servitude, (4) right to education, and (5) right to treatment. R. A. Burt and O. M. Fiss, *Hierarchy and Value* (unpublished seminar materials, Spring, 1981) at 32.

3. The Pennsylvania School Code of 1949, Section 1304, provided: "The board of school directors of any school district may refuse to accept or retain beginners who have not attained a mental age of five years, as determined by the supervisor of special education or a . . . public school psychologist." And the Pennsylvania School Code of 1949, Section 1375, provided: "Uneducable children provided for by Department of Public Welfare . . . [which shall] arrange for the care, training and supervision of such child in a manner not inconsistent with the laws governing mentally defective individuals."

4. 347 U.S. 483, 495 (U.S. 1954) For an account of *Brown v. Board of Education* and the systematic litigation strategy that resulted in overthrowing *de jure* segregation in schools, see Richard Kluger, *Simple Justice: A History of Brown v. Board of Education and Black America's Struggle for Equality* (New York: Alfred Knopf, 1976).

5. 347 U.S. at 493.

6. *Id.*

7. 343 F. Supp. 279 (E.D. Pa. 1972).

8. 343 F. Supp. at 283 n. 8. The court found it necessary to reach the Equal Protection claim because Intermediate Units that objected to the settlement had challenged the court's subject-matter jurisdiction. 343 F. Supp. at 289, 293 ff.

9. The court noted that beginning in 1912, the Research Section of the Eugenic Society, known as the American Breeders' Association, suggested that segregation and other "drastic measures" needed to be taken to protect American society from the menace of "the feebleminded." 343 F. Supp. at 294.

10. 343 F. Supp. at 284. The court noted that in the early twentieth century, special education classes for children with intellectual disabilities were denominated "opportunity classes," indicating that the child was simply waiting to join the mainstream of the school, but that in the next decade they became "dumping grounds for children who could not manage in other classes." 343 F. Supp. at 294.

11. P.L. 94–142.

12. 20 U.S.C. 1401 *et seq.*

13. Section 5. Fourteenth Amendment to the United States Constitution.

14. Pub. L. No. 94–142, § 3(a), 89 Stat. 775 (1975) (codified at 20 U.S.C. 1400(b)(9) (1988)); see also S. Rep. No. 168, 94th Cong., 1st Sess. 13, 22 (1975); H. R. Rep. No. 332, 94th Cong., 1st Sess. 14 (1975). When Congress reenacted IDEA in 1997, it retained this finding—see 20 U.S.C. 1400(c)(6)—and explained that it wished "to restate that the 'right to equal educational opportunities' is inherent in the equal protection clause of the 14th Amendment to the U.S. Constitution." S. Rep. No. 275, 104th Cong., 2d Sess. 31 (1996).

15. See https://teachingamericanhistory.org/library/document/speech-on-the-dred-scott-decision.

16. 29 U.S.C. § 794; https://www.eeoc.gov/laws/statutes/rehab.cfm.

17. 42 U.S.C. 12101 *et seq.*; https://www.ada.gov/ada_intro.htm.

18. Humphrey v. Cady, 405 U.S. 504, 509 (U.S. 1972).

19. See O'Connor v. Donaldson, 422 U.S. 563, 580, 95 S. Ct. 2486, 45 L. Ed. 2d 396 (1975) (Burger, C. J., concurring).

20. 364 U.S. 479, 5 L. Ed. 2d 231, 81 S. Ct. 247 (1960).

21. In Shelton, the Court struck down an Arkansas statute that required every teacher to file an annual affidavit listing all organizations to which he or she belonged or contributed.

22. 437 F. Supp. 1209, 1216 (E.D. La. 1976).

23. 404 F. Supp. 430 (M.D. Tenn. 1974).

24. 442 U.S. 584 (U.S. 1979).

25. 406 U.S. 715, 737, 32 L. Ed. 2d 435, 92 S. Ct. 1845.

26. 422 U.S. 563, 576, 45 L. Ed. 2d 396, 95 S. Ct. 2486.

27. 522 F. Supp. 171, 239 (D.N.H. 1981).

28. *Id.*, citing O'Connor v. Donaldson, 422 U.S. at 574, n.9.

29. *Id.*, citing Rogers v. Okin, 634 F.2d 650, 657 (1st Cir. 1980).

30. Morton Birnbaum, "The Right to Treatment," *Journal of the American Bar Association* 46 (1960): 499–505.

31. 46 A.B.A.J. at 503.

32. 373 F.2d 451, 452, 453, 455 (D.C. Cir. 1966).

33. 503 F.2d 1305, 1312 (5th Cir. 1974).

34. 437 F. Supp. 1209, 1219 (E.D. La. 1976).

35. See Roy G. Spece, "Preserving the Right to Treatment: A Critical Assessment and Constructive Development of Constitutional Right to Treatment Theories," *Arizona Law Review* 20, no. 1 (1978), citing Donaldson v. O'Connor, 493 F.2d 507, 520–25 (5th Cir. 1974), vacated on other grounds and remanded, 422 U.S. 563 (1975).

36. 357 F. Supp. 752, 761 (E.D. N.Y. 1973).

37. See Dandridge v. Williams, 397 U.S. 471, 487, 90 S. Ct. 1153, 1163, 25 L. Ed. 2d 491 (1970) (holding that the Constitution does not empower a court to "second-guess state officials charged with the difficult responsibility of allocating limited public welfare funds among the myriad of potential recipients").

38. See In re Gault, 387 U.S. 1, 22 n. 30 (1967).

39. See Donaldson v. O'Connor, 493 F.2d at 522 n. 21.

40. See, for example, Rone v. Fireman, 473 F. Supp. 92, 119 (N.D. Ohio 1979).

41. Ibid., 85.

42. See Spece, *supra*, at 8–9.

43. See Jonas Robitscher, "The Right to Psychiatric Treatment: A Social-Legal Approach to the Plight of the State Hospital Patient," *Villanova Law Review* 18 (November 1972): 11–36, https://digitalcommons.law.villanova.edu/cgi/viewcontent.cgi?article=1956&context=vlr.

44. 446 F. Supp. at 1318.

45. *Id.*

46. 370 U.S. 660, 8 L. Ed. 2d 758, 82 S. Ct. 1417 (1962).

47. 373 F. Supp. 487, 496 (D. Minn. 1974), *aff'd*, 550 F.2d 1122 (8th Cir. 1977).

48. 370 U.S. 660, 676, 82 S. Ct. 1417, 8 L. Ed. 2d 758 (Douglas, J., concurring).

49. *Id.* at 496.

50. 357 F. Supp. 752, 764 (E.D. N.Y. 1973).

51. *Id.* at 764–65.

52. 357 F. Supp. at 761–65.

53. 430 U.S. 651, 664–48 (1977).

54. *Id.* at 669 n. 37.

55. In re Joyce Z., 4 D&C 3d 597 (Allegheny Co. 1975).

56. Michael Kindred, "Beyond the Right to Habilitation," in *The Mentally Retarded Citizen and the Law* (New York: Free Press, 1975), 425–32.

57. 29 U.S.C. § 793.

58. 446 F. Supp. at 1323.

59. *Id.* at 1323–24.

60. See, for example, Garrity v. Gallen, 522 F. Supp. 171 (D.N.H. 1981); Homeward Bound v. The Hissom Memorial Center, No. 85-C-437-E (N.D. Okla. July 24, 1987); Jackson v. Fort Stanton Hospital and Training School, 757 F. Supp 1243 (D.N.M. 1990).

61. 42 U.S.C. § 12101.

62. 42 U.S.C. § 12101(a)(2).

63. 28 U.S.C. § 35.130(b)(1)(iv).

64. 527 U.S. 581 (1999).

65. *Id.*, 527 U.S. at 597.

66. *Id.*, 527 U.S. at 587.

67. 527 U.S. at 602, quoting 42 U.S.C. 12131(2).

CHAPTER 7

# The Rise of Self-Advocacy

## *A Personal Remembrance*

MARK FRIEDMAN AND NANCY K. NOWELL

*Note: This chapter contains the individual recollections of two leaders in the advocacy movement.*

Like many residents, Jerome Iannuzzi Jr. came to Pennhurst State School and Hospital as a child. In surprising ways, his life came to embody the spirit of self-determination and self-advocacy. His would be a personal "freedom struggle" that opened the door for many. Little did Jerome know when he first took that long drive onto Pennhurst's sprawling and secluded compound that he would experience the fruits of his own liberation as a spokesman for so many others who walked a similar path.

Jerome was only thirteen years of age when he and his brother arrived in 1951. During his long stay, Jerome saw and experienced many kinds of abuse and moments of terror. He was forced to work for no pay on the farms that grew the food that fellow residents consumed each day. At night he fed, showered, and cleaned residents who were referred to as "low functioning." While at Pennhurst, a caring staff person taught him the basics of reading and writing.

Jerome was released in 1966 at age twenty-eight. By 1985, he had become one of the early leaders in the self-advocacy movement and an officer of Speaking for Ourselves (SFO). He worked tirelessly for his friends and colleagues still living in institutions. Jerome made presentations to governmental officials, college students, and professional groups. When we first started doing work to close institutions, he was worried about the folks with the most severe disabilities. He would say, "Where are they going to go?" He knew firsthand how much help some people needed, and it was hard for him to fully embrace community life for everyone. He had to go visit several homes in the community and see some of the people he had provided care for at the institution now living successfully in the community. After that, he became a fierce advocate for everyone to live in the community.

In 1990, Jerome was appointed by Governor Dick Thornburgh to serve on the Pennsylvania Developmental Disabilities Council. This gave him a platform to speak out against the institutions and promote their closure. He was one of the first self-advocates in the country to be appointed in his own right to serve on a Developmental Disabilities Council. Jerome spoke at public forums of his experience as "a frightened child locked in a room" and about "seeing the unmarked graves of people who had lived almost their whole lives at Pennhurst."

Jerome shocked everyone in 1993 when he announced his marriage engagement to Carole Talley, who was also a member of Speaking for Ourselves. Other advocates had not known that they had been longtime sweethearts at Pennhurst. At that time, few former residents of institutions had gotten married. Many of Jerome's friends and advocacy colleagues were genuinely worried about the idea of them being married. Several approached me in disbelief that the marriage would work, saying, "Mark, you have to do something about this." I finally found the answer to their unsupportive questions and replied, "Jerome should have the same opportunity to mess up his relationships just like most of us have." That put a stop to the discussion. They had a lovely wedding ceremony with dozens of their friends attending. Carole was a vision of splendor in the handmade wedding gown designed and constructed by a friend, who was also one of the principal attorneys in the *Pennhurst* case. That seamstress was attorney and author Judith Gran.

Not long after the wedding, Jerome shocked us again when he announced he could no longer be an advocate and that he was even giving up serving on the Developmental Disabilities Council, a position he dearly loved. When asked, he astonished his friends by saying he was married now and had to take care of his wife, Carole. "That's what you do, Mark," he said, "When you get married." Ten years later when we all celebrated their ten-year wedding anniversary together, I realized he had certainly been right about how to have a loving marriage.

In 2003, television reporter Bill Baldini (see chapter 4) did a follow-up news segment about Pennhurst, with a special appearance by Jerome and Carole. When Baldini asked Carole how she felt about being in the community and married to Jerome, she cried, "It's like Heaven!" Jerome passed away at the end of the year in 2003 from a heart condition. The advocacy movement had lost a powerful voice for freedom and justice.

## The Pennhurst Legacy of Self-Advocacy

The Pennhurst lawsuits and its closure in 1987 were instrumental to the rise of the self-advocacy movement in America. Speaking for Ourselves and other organized self-advocacy groups changed the entire landscape of public policy and practice in the disability movement.

At the time Speaking for Ourselves was formed in 1982, people with intellectual and developmental disabilities were one of the most oppressed groups in society. They were very dependent on staff and families for meeting their everyday needs. While progress was being made in terms of services and supports, most of the stigma and prejudices had not changed. As such, people with developmental disabilities were perceived to be incapable of advocating for themselves. Most decisions were made for people rather than empowering the person to make or learn how to make their own decisions.

The self-advocacy movement—former residents speaking from their own experiences—would fundamentally test and ultimately change those perceptions. It shifted the balance of power from professionals and parents toward the people themselves, just as other movements of oppressed peoples had done before. But to do so, people had to overcome their lack of money, limited access to telephones, illiteracy, inability to drive, and other resources that most people took for granted in the twentieth century. People would have to learn to overcome their lack of experiences and skills. That they were able to successfully do so is due to their resiliency and perseverance. This is the essence of self-determination.

This story is told largely in the first person through the medium of oral history, and it includes the memories of the facilitator/coordinator and the words of key leaders of Speaking for Ourselves.

## How Did Speaking for Ourselves Get Started?

I began working for the Pennhurst Special Master on October 1, 1978, as an intern while I was finishing my master's degree in organizational development. The Special Master's office was an arm of the U.S. Federal Court, set up to oversee implementation of the Pennhurst Court Order.[1] Our office was in King of Prussia, Pennsylvania.

In October 1980, I saw for the first time the film *People First*[2] at a monthly staff meeting. The film was a documentary about People First of Oregon, the first self-advocacy group to be formed in the United States. The film showed the first statewide conference of People First, held in Salem, Oregon, in October 1974. It showed people coming to the conference and people with significant disabilities speaking up. I was moved to tears by the film and the notion that people who were perceived to be voiceless could gain a voice and could be organizing and could be in charge of having their own conference.

Afterward, I was startled to realize that no one else in the room had been so affected by the film. The film was like a personal message sent directly to me. Seeing the film inspired me to help start a similar self-advocacy group in Pennsylvania, which eventually would become the statewide self-advocacy organization called Speaking for Ourselves. It was the *People First* film that motivated me to take action. Much later, I would learn that at the same time people with developmental disabilities were planning the first self-advocacy conference ever held in America; in October 1974 disability advocates were filing the landmark *Pennhurst* lawsuit in federal court.

In 1980, there were only four or five states around the country that had self-advocacy organizations, and I thought at the time, how could it be that there were no self-advocacy groups in Pennsylvania? The Commonwealth had one of the largest networks of Community Living Arrangement programs in the country. Pennsylvania was perceived nationally to have many cutting-edge services. If there were so many "cutting-edge" services, why was there no self-advocacy association? It would take me years to understand that having a well-developed service system was the biggest barrier to the development of self-advocacy.

Families and providers were very resistant to the notion that the people themselves could speak up on their own behalf. Often it was necessary for them to step aside and allow people to develop their own voice. Many advocates and professionals were not very open to stepping aside or to working with us. They didn't see it in their self-interest to have people with disabilities speak up. It was a tough nut to crack. Fortunately, at the time, I had no idea how hard the task would be. I was naïve and didn't realize the many barriers that would have to be overcome. I didn't appreciate how strongly the entrenched interests would resist the development of self-advocacy.

Finally, in late 1981, I decided that we needed to take some action. I went to the local Montgomery County Arc and spoke to somebody I knew there. They gave me a room and invited people from a local sheltered workshop to attend a meeting to discuss creating a self-advocacy group. Five people showed up (Harry Cappuccio, Lynn Armbrust, Luann Carter, Domenic Rossi, and Sarah Brown). I had no idea what I was doing. In fact, I'd never been in a room with five people with disabilities, let alone asking them for their ideas. However, I was an experienced group facilitator, and I had done a lot of organizing work as part of the Vietnam antiwar movement. I had the skills, knowledge, and understanding of how you bring people together.

I showed the *People First* film, and the group's reaction was very surprising to me. One of the participants who lived in a group home said, "Mark, that movie is sad. Those people are so disabled." I was very surprised that the film, which I had found so inspiring, fell flat on the group. But everyone was interested in the idea of putting on their own conference. We began holding weekly meetings to plan the conference for 1982. The Montgomery County Arc donated space, and we met weekly for five weeks in their offices in an old, rundown former mansion.

One of the really fascinating things was how we chose the name Speaking for Ourselves. At that time, most groups that existed were called People First. From an organizing perspective, I wanted to use that name because the words were very powerful and would link us to other efforts, but the group had no interest in those words. The group was very hesitant regarding the use of words and labels to define them, but we did need language to use in the conference invitation. Finally, I said, "Okay, I know everybody hates this word but what are you going do about this mental retardation word?" They all turned on me and Sarah Brown said, "Mark, that's a terrible thing to say." I felt like a knife had gone through my heart because I was supposed to be the good guy.

The group talked about being called that dirty word in school when they would get on the school bus and just how painful it was. Finally, I told the group I understood, but they had to come up with some words to use. They had to write an invitation. If they didn't like the bad words, they still had to come up with something they did like. The group started with, "We're inviting 'people like ourselves' to come to this conference." Eventually, over time that sentiment evolved into Speaking for Ourselves. When asked why that name was chosen, Roland Johnson, a key leader, said, "Oh, can't you see it? What we call ourselves is what we do."[3]

After the success of the first conference, we were unclear how to proceed. Luann Carter, the group's founder, and I were invited to attend the next annual conference of People First of Oregon where the *People First* film was made. Rick Robinson, a staff member of the Arc, Montgomery County, worked tirelessly to obtain free airplane tickets from the airline to enable us to attend. Luann says of the event, "I was overwhelmed by the size of the group, one thousand people, and how it was run. When I got there, I asked them, didn't they have a place for me to speak as I had traveled so far? I was allowed to speak in front of the entire conference and told them what a real pleasure it was to be invited. They were real supportive and caring in the way they helped everyone out."[4]

Over the next six months we developed five local chapters. The first chapter presidents included: Steve Dorsey, Roland Johnson, Louis Newburg, Richard Humor, and Karen Hayes. The group traveled across the state to Harrisburg and Pittsburgh to start chapters, but they fell through in spite of much effort. At that time, I had been laid off from my prior job, and I was doing this as a volunteer. I worked like a madman traveling every night to different chapter meetings and organizing during the day. People would ask me where had we gotten the funding to get started? I would tell them I had a government grant, and they would ask with great curiosity, "Where did you get it?" as they were interested in doing the same, and, I would tell them—*unemployment insurance*. In a manner of speaking, the government was paying me to help start Speaking for Ourselves. By then, I was working full-time as a volunteer for the organization.

In the first few years, members would attend local chapter meetings and raise issues such as problems they were having with their roommate. Other chapter members would give suggestions on how they might handle it. As members began to gain their voice, they began to bring up problems they were having with their providers. As such, the chapters became safe zones where members could speak up freely and gain support from each other. Domenic Rossi, the first president of Speaking for Ourselves, had a chapter rule: "What's said here, stays here."

Each chapter had one or two volunteer advisors and many supporters who assisted by providing rides, food money, attendant care, advice, and support. The chapter advisors played key roles in providing support and guidance to the chapter officers as they developed the leadership skills to run their own organization. The advisor contribution was largely that of a community organizer; they helped chapter members' work collectively together to gain strength and build their own organization. The advisor role was frequently misunderstood. This was primarily because unlike other movements, self-advocacy was situated in a human service environment whose main role was to provide protection and care rather than a social justice perspective working to enhance freedom and self-determination.

Over time, as the chapters built strength in numbers, they began to take collective action. We had meetings with governmental officials to attempt to resolve individual issues. We began inviting powerful governmental officials to be speakers at our local chapters to meet people and hear their concerns directly. I would later learn that many of the original state self-advocacy organizations developed in the same manner.[5]

Prominent officials attended the local chapter meetings, including Congressman Peter Kostmayer, State Representatives Joe Hoeffel and John Fox, Senator John Heinz, and the governor's wife, Ginny Thornburgh. She visited and spoke at our local chapter meeting at the Montgomery County Public Library. I can still remember the football fullback–sized security agent who remained standing in the back of the library the entire time. The governor and Mrs. Thornburgh had a child with disabilities, and she was very active in this area. They became important allies and their involvement opened doors for self-advocacy.

In 1985, we were successful in getting Jerome Iannuzzi, one of the early leaders of Speaking for Ourselves, appointed by Governor Dick Thornburgh to serve on the Pennsylvania Developmental Disabilities Council. I had been appointed to the DD Council previously and was able to get Jerome appointed initially to a council committee and later to the full council. Jerome was a pioneer. He was one of the first self-advocates in the country to be appointed in his own right to serve on a DD Council.

Jerome had lived at Pennhurst State School and Hospital for more than fifteen years as a child and young adult. He explained his reason for being at Pennhurst this way: "When I was 13, my parents decided their lives would be better if I was cared for in an institution. Although an aunt and uncle wanted to adopt me, the Judge said no, and I was committed to Pennhurst. Today, I wish families and the government could be institutionalized and see how it feels for themselves."[6]

Jerome was a tireless disabilities rights advocate and leader who never forgot the people living in institutions. He fought his whole life to help people get out of institutions. Throughout his advocacy career, Jerome made hundreds of public presentations to governmental officials, college students, professionals, and the general public, advocating for the rights of people with disabilities to live in the community. He was a frequent participant on local radio stations and interviewed for local newspapers.

As the members of Speaking for Ourselves began to speak up more forcefully, the leaders began working to address these in a more systematic manner. The annual conferences began to address more significant issues. Issues people talked about were transportation, relationships, group homes, institutions, and sheltered workshops. After institutions, sheltered workshops were the biggest issue the members talked and complained about. The majority of the members were attending sheltered workshops daily. In the sheltered workshops people earned twenty to fifty cents *an hour*. It was hard to believe. People would actually show me their paycheck to prove that they had only received $2.65 or $12.54 for five days of work. Sheltered workshops became the first systemic advocacy issue the group chose to address by embracing the positive notion of "We want jobs."

In 1985, in conjunction with the Temple University Institute on Disabilities, we conducted an evaluation of a local sheltered workshop. Five self-advocates were hired to work as project consultants, and they designed the survey questions and interviewed more than one hundred people who worked in the workshop. This was the first time that people with intellectual disabilities had served as the researchers and conducted the interview themselves. There was so much skepticism that people with intellectual disabilities could serve as researchers that we had to prove reliability. We tape recorded all of the interviews and had the answer sheets compared with the tape recordings by a third party.

An extremely interesting finding from the evaluation was that 93 percent of the people reported they liked working in the workshop and at the same time 80 percent wanted to get a job outside of the workshop. The results of the project were later published in a peer-reviewed scientific journal.[7] Two years later we carried out another contract to conduct interviews for a research project. We interviewed sixty-eight people who had jobs in supported employment demonstration programs across the state about their job satisfaction. This time, no one demanded we prove reliability.

Betty Potts was one of the people who worked on the Temple interview projects. Betty was a young African American woman who had never learned to read. To participate in the project, Betty had to memorize a half-page introduction to be said at the beginning of each interview. Twenty-five years later, she can still recite that introduction from memory. Betty had lived at Pennhurst and was the first person to move out under the federal court's ruling and orders in 1978. She became a key leader in Speaking for Ourselves and in 1984 attended the very first International People First Conference in Seattle, Washington.

Entering Pennhurst at age thirteen, Betty left in 1978 at the age of twenty-two. She had lived in North Philadelphia with her parents but when her parents could no longer take care of her she was sent to the institution. In Betty's own words, she described her life at Pennhurst:

> I went to Pennhurst when I was nine. I got sent there because my Mom was getting sick and she couldn't take care of me. I remember being at Pennhurst and seeing people tied down to their beds and getting smacked and hit. Nobody hit me 'cause I could talk. I once spoke up about their hitting someone and handled rough, but they said I lied about it, but I didn't.
>
> It was hard living at Pennhurst. I guess it was also hard on the staff 'cause some of them were overworked. My mom and dad didn't put me there because they didn't love me. They put me there 'cause they couldn't take care of me. I always went home to visit with my dad and mom even though I was living at Pennhurst.
>
> At Pennhurst, I lived in a dormitory with a whole bunch of beds on each side. When I got to be an adult, I lived in a training ward and I used to feed the other kids 'cause they couldn't feed themselves. I loved feeding them and helping out. I still see two of them today. When I first went to Pennhurst, I wasn't in a wheelchair and I could walk using a walker.
>
> When I got out, the first house I moved to was [a] group home. I was walking then with a crutch, before I needed a wheelchair, and there was a bit of a problem because the house had a step up to the entrance and it wasn't easy to get up, but I did it. I had two roommates

> and we went to the supermarket together. We had a list and we were picking out the food.
>
> One time, right after I got out of Pennhurst, I was having behavioral problems, throwing stuff. When you see people banging their head against the wall and throwing stuff and lots of people getting attention, you start doing it, too.
>
> Then I got a behavioral therapist, and she told me if I didn't have those behaviors, I could get my own apartment. It was the best thing I ever worked for. You don't know what it's like to have your own place. You don't have other people around screaming or bothering you. I had a boyfriend for a while after I got out, but he started to talk about having a baby and I said babies need a lot of care, so he went his way and I went mine.[8]

In 1986, Speaking for Ourselves chose employment for its next conference, entitled "Real Jobs in the Community." We received several complaints from professionals who claimed we were insulting people working in sheltered workshops by suggesting that they did not have real jobs. However, none of the members complained. For them, working in a sheltered workshop for piece rate and subminimum wage was not a real job. The conference sessions were cofacilitated by supported work job coaches and people in supported work. The conference was planned by many of the initial founders of Speaking for Ourselves. Their thoughts and concerns about employment included:

- "At a real job, you work eight hours a day and you get paid for it. You have responsibility. But in the workshop, they always tell you 'you can't do it.'" —Jerome Iannuzzi
- "In the workshop, they are supposed to help you get out and get a real job—but they don't. They always say I'm 'not ready'—but I am." —Peggy Carney
- "There's only one good thing you can say about working in a workshop—it's better than staying at home going stir-crazy." —Domenic Rossi
- "We need more learning and training than we are getting in the workshop." —Harry Cappuccio and Lynn Armbrust

Robert Perske, a nationally famous disability writer, was one of the conference speakers. He requested to speak at the close of the conference so he could reflect on what he had seen and experienced. In his speech, he talked about self-advocacy being a *movement*, and he said a movement needs its own music. Unbeknownst to us, Karl Williams, a local singer/songwriter, was in the audience. Karl later told us that when he heard that sentence he said to himself: I am a songwriter, I know how to write songs. Karl worked with us and took the words we said and put them in a song, titled "Speaking for Ourselves." In 1987, fifteen of the members packed into a professional sound studio and recorded the song. It later became the unofficial anthem of the self-advocacy movement and has been sung and adopted by groups around the world.

### Sexual Abuse and Assault: The Fellowship Farm Retreat

For several years, we had held an annual leadership retreat for all of the chapter officers and boards of directors. We had about fifty people attend a weekend event at Fellowship Farm, a rural retreat center located not far from the Pennhurst campus. During the third retreat, a leader asked SFO to contribute a chapter to a new book. Anyone that was interested in participating met after dinner. General questions were asked that related to the focus of the chapter. One advisor asked the group, "Has anyone ever been hurt by a staff member?" The next four hours changed Speaking for Ourselves and everyone in the room forever.

Every member in the room had a story of physical and/or sexual abuse. When one person stopped talking another would start. As advisors we felt completely overwhelmed and had no idea how to manage the amount of pain that encompassed everyone in the room. Each story made it easier for the next person to talk, but harder and harder to hear. The group finally ended, but the flashbacks, crying, and PTSD symptoms that we had inadvertently triggered continued through the night and into the next day.

That experience marked a sea change for the organization and its members. As advisors we knew we had been given a gift. It had taken two years for members to share with us this most private part of their lives. They spoke of stories of rape, incest, and physical brutality. Many had been raped multiple times by the same person or by different people. The perpetrators were not just staff—they were siblings, stepfathers, uncles, neighbors, bus drivers, and many times other people with disabilities.

We had a great responsibility to listen and honor the pain that they shared with us. We believed them and put support and counseling resources in place to help them process their trauma. After that retreat, every Speaking for Ourselves conference had at least one session dedicated to talking about sexual assault. One of the advisors changed the focus of her career to start working with victims of sexual assault who have disabilities.[9]

By the late 1980s, Speaking for Ourselves was becoming better known around the country. We spoke at conferences in New York, Virginia, Ohio, Tennessee, Illinois, Wisconsin, Texas, Colorado, and Washington, and internationally, in London, England. We made presentations at most of the national disability conferences, including TASH, American Association for Mental Retardation, and the Arc of the United States. Members participated in rallies in Harrisburg and Philadelphia to advocate for community services. We networked with national advocacy leaders like Justin Dart, Ginny Thornburgh, and numerous state legislators. We testified in federal court and to the United States Congress in Washington, D.C., and to Pennsylvania governmental officials in Harrisburg. We helped the National Park Service make Independence Hall more accessible. We worked with the League of Women Voters on voter registration.

## The Institution Campaign

The infamous Pennhurst state institution closed in 1987. Roland Johnson, former resident of Pennhurst and board president of Speaking for Ourselves, had been a keynote speaker at the closing ceremony and interviewed on the WHYY radio station by a well-known radio personality, Marty Moss-Coane, in 1987.[10] Despite the closure of Pennhurst and other state institutions, tens of thousands of people still lived in segregated facilities. Roland Johnson and many of our members who had lived at Pennhurst and other institutions felt the hurt and pain personally.

It took several years for people to be able to talk about their institution experiences. Many members had lived in institutions, and most had had experiences of physical and/or sexual assault. It was very hard to talk about, and many never did. People's feelings about their experience in institutions were complicated. In general, they included: (1) feeling abandoned by their families and not wanting to talk bad about them, (2) living in fear, (3) recalling the actual experience of abuse, and (4) experiencing the lingering feelings of shame and fear. These feelings were compounded by a sense that "it must have been my fault," "I must have done something bad to have been put there." Almost everyone who had lived in an institution had tremendous fear that they would be sent back. These fears were often played upon by group home staff, who would threaten people by saying things like, "If you don't behave, you will be sent back to Pennhurst."

Nonetheless, slowly and over time people began more and more to talk about institutions. The issue was usually addressed as a question similar to, "How can we help all the people still living in institutions?" "What can we do to help them get out?"

Speaking for Ourselves began an effort to get people out of institutions, first by simply visiting people still living in such facilities. We had taken the position not to have local chapters in state institutions and instead worked to get the people living in the institutions to attend local chapter meetings. We had members who had been in in three state institutions attending the chapter meetings. Debbie Robinson was the Philadelphia chapter president and remembers: "They came to us telling us things and told us to come to see them, and to get them out. One of the members just stood out and said come visit me. That's when we went to this institution."

State officials didn't want us visiting the institutions, but they could not stop us from visiting our members who lived there. On one of our first visits to Woodhaven Center, we were told we could not go onto the living unit where our members lived "because it is an infringement on the rights of the other residents."

On another occasion, Jerome Iannuzzi, an SFO officer and a former resident of Pennhurst, and I were visiting people living at Embreeville State Center, another Pennsylvania state institution. Our inspection unearthed many advocacy concerns. On the way home in the car, we were discussing the next steps we would take, and he said, "Mark, I can't do this anymore." I said, "What do you mean?" He said he couldn't visit the institutions anymore. It was just too difficult because it brought up all his own past painful experiences.

Jerome would later become a pioneer again, when he married his long-time sweetheart, Carole Talley. They had met when they both lived in Pennhurst. They married in 1993, and in 2003 they celebrated their ten-year wedding anniversary with a large party with many friends at their side. Theirs was the first of the many romances that emerged over time from Speaking for Ourselves. Carole had also lived at Pennhurst and that was where they first met. Carole discussed her life at Pennhurst and other institutions:

> You people don't know what it's like to be in an institution. When I was three years old, I was taken from my family. My family didn't have a choice. They didn't have the money. I grew up in Elwyn for twenty-three years and in plain words, they ain't no damn good.
>
> I feel everybody on earth has a right to live where they want to live, not in an institution. I feel [bad] every time people mention the word retarded; I get very angry because I hate that word. They should use the word disabled.
>
> I feel all institutions should be closed for good. I wish that families and government officials could be in an institution to see how it is for themselves. I lived in three of them and I can tell you how it was. They were no fun to be in. When I was two years old, my doctor examined me and did not expect me to live. I kept going back and forth to doctors. My parents did without many things because of the medical bills. I walked into the table and they found out I had a tumor on my brain and my parents had to put me away. I had water on the brain and a tumor pressing against my nerves. They had to take it out using needles. I thought I was going insane.

> They put me in an institution. My grandfather wanted me but my mom said no. When I went to the institution, they told my parents they would teach me reading, writing, and arithmetic but they did not teach me anything. They left me alone in a classroom, and a couple of boys got a hold of me and raped me. When my mom left, the other kids beat me up. When you have an accident, they would make you kneel on the floor and put your hands out and put the dirty panties over your face. Every time my mom would come to see me she could see marks. When she would say something, I would get beat up and put in the locked side room. Every five minutes I was in the side room. My parents couldn't visit me.
>
> I could tell you about three institutions I lived in: Elwyn, Pennhurst, and Woodhaven. I really feel that I was left out in the cold, because people called me names and labeled me retarded. I wish people would refer to us as disabled.[11]

Roland Johnson, the president of the board of directors and a former resident of Pennhurst led what became the Campaign for Freedom. He was a fearless advocate who became a national leader of the self-advocacy movement. Roland would later have his life story of what he called "living in a desert world" published as a major book, *Lost in a Desert World*.[12] His accomplishments were widely recognized through the disability rights community and the larger political culture.[13]

In 1989, we visited a local one-hundred-bed private institution that had previously been called Pennhurst Annex. While there, Roland heard a staff person slap a resident. At the institution, we met several small children who spent their whole day confined to their beds. Roland came out in the hallway and said, "Mark, there are babies being kept there." Debbie described her experience, "I was stunned, I was dumbfounded and I've never seen anything like it in my life. There were no words you could say besides the smell in there. It made me sick. I've never seen anything like it." We called everyone we knew, including the Arc state director and lawyers. We met with Commonwealth officials about the horrible conditions at the facility. An investigation was done and the state sent in monitors at the facility 24/7. We visited this facility many times and had many meetings with officials about the awful conditions, but in the end little was done.

## The ADA Signing

Justin Dart, considered the "father" of the Americans with Disabilities Act (ADA), invited Speaking for Ourselves to attend the bill signing ceremony at the White House by President George H. W. Bush in 1990. Roland Johnson, Steve Dorsey, Debbie Robinson, and I were able to attend.[14]

We reserved an inexpensive hotel in downtown Washington, D.C., for the night before the big event. When we arrived, the hotel was in disarray from a major water leak. They told us they had made alternative overnight arrangements for us at a hotel down the street and that we should just drive over there. They pointed at an office building across the street. We were quite anxious of what we might find. We drove up a driveway of a high-rise building and around a corner and there, seemingly out of nowhere, appeared two doormen. It was a hotel entrance. The doormen were attired in high-topped leather boots, long waistcoats, and top hats. "Welcome to the Watergate," they said. We were about to stay overnight at the famous and posh Watergate Hotel that was at the heart of the Watergate break-in in the 1970s that led to President Nixon's resignation.

It was a very expensive hotel, but we were not charged anything above the rate we had already paid. The rooms had exquisite old-fashioned furniture and thick, luxurious white bathrobes, which Roland quickly wrapped himself in. I told the doorman we were going to the White House for the ADA ceremony the next day and asked how we could get there. He said just come down to the lobby in the morning and the staff would make arrangements for us. So, we all arose early the next morning and came down to the lobby and asked for a cab to be called. Up pulled a limo. The doorman said it was part of the Watergate hotel service and we were transported to the front gate of the White House in style.

The ADA signing ceremony was very moving to all of us. Debbie Robinson described it in this way:

> Well, it was hotter than I can imagine. In July, you don't want to be on D.C. It was one of the hottest things I have ever seen, sitting in the sun just waiting, I mean we were, I don't know how long, two or three hours. It was really hot that day. It was the most incredible thing I have ever seen. I don't know how to describe something, you see the President of the United States and you see this man in a wheelchair with a hat. How did Justin [Dart] do it all? It was the most incredible thing I have ever seen to meet the man that went all over the country to work on this.
>
> Justin came around to meet us in the hot sun. There were no words that you could describe, something you can't say it. There is nothing I could say or I was frozen in time or something 'cause you never met an icon. It was like meeting the greatest leader in time, a whole lot like Martin Luther King or Gandhi. It was just incredible.[15]

## Forming the National Self-Advocacy Organization

We had been working with other state self-advocacy organizations for several years. We wanted to form a national self-advocacy organization as a means to gain strength and to learn from each other. In May 1990, we attended an American Association for Mental Retardation (AAMR) national conference in Atlanta Georgia that had set aside space to hold a self-advocacy forum. Jerome Iannuzzi and I attended the meeting, and forming a national association was discussed.

At the meeting, we met representatives from People First of Tennessee. We had a lot in common with them as they were also working on institution issues. They would ultimately file two federal lawsuits on behalf of their members living in state institutions in response to horrendous conditions and multiple deaths in Tennessee institutions. They were the only self-advocacy organization to ever file a successful lawsuit against state institutions.

In 1990, we sent five of our board officers to the First National Self-Advocacy Conference held in Estes Park, outside Denver, Colorado. The officers had been authorized by the Speaking for Ourselves Board of Directors to form a national organization. At that meeting, Debbie Robinson and Roland Johnson led the discussion and a national steering committee was formed to pursue the idea.

The following year, 1991, the Second National Self-Advocacy Conference was held in Nashville, Tennessee. The work of the steering committee was presented and the eight hundred attendees voted to create Self-Advocates Becoming Empowered (SABE). Roland Johnson became an officer and leader of SABE.

In 1993, Roland would give the most famous speech of his life, entitled, "Who's in Control?" at the Third International People First Conference in Toronto, Canada.[16] The hall was filled with more than one thousand self-advocates from twenty-two countries around the world. Roland's words rang out loud and clear across the huge hotel ballroom. "Who's in control?" he shouted. "I want to know are you in control or are staff in control?" "We are, we are," the audience yelled over and over. "Who's in charge over you? Are you in charge? Is staff in charge?" "No, no, no," yelled the audience. "But who's in charge?" bellowed Roland. "We are," came yells from the audience. Finally, Roland led the audience in, "I want to be in charge of my own life, can you say that with me?" And the audience responded loudly. One of the first issues SABE chose to address was institutions. This led to a national campaign that was carried out by state self-advocacy associations across the country.

In 1995, the singer/songwriter Karl Williams wrote the "Close the Doors" song in association with SABE and we were able to record it together in a recording studio. The lyrics are included in the postscript at the end of this chapter.

Later that year, we participated in a joint meeting of self-advocates from around the country with the U.S. Justice Department in Washington, D.C. The Justice Department had filed numerous lawsuits against state institutions under the Civil Rights of Institutionalized Persons Act (CRIPA). However, they frequently settled the lawsuits by agreeing to court orders to fix up the institution rather than having people move out into community programs. We met with Deval Patrick, the assistant attorney general for the Civil Rights Division of the Department of Justice (and later governor of Massachusetts). Pam Bard, our Chester County chapter president, spoke forcefully to Mr. Patrick, demanding to know what he personally was going to do about all the people still living in institutions.

In July 1997, we jointly planned and participated in a national retreat at Wingspread Retreat Center in Minneapolis, Minnesota, as part of Self-Advocates Becoming Empowered. The Close the Doors Campaign to close all the institutions in the United States was officially launched at this event.

Along with the national campaign, we continued our state institution work by visiting institutions and speaking out against them constantly and consistently. The state Protection and Advocacy director, Ilene Shane, later said, "We were always on message." She said that whenever she was in a meeting where members of Speaking for Ourselves were present, they would always ask her—What was she doing about institutions?

We conducted our Campaign for Freedom and visited all of the seven state institutions in Pennsylvania. We traveled across the state because many of the institutions are in the remote corners of the state. In 1997, the Pennsylvania State Legislature proposed a law restricting the ability of the governor to close an institution without legislative approval. State Representative Fairchild chaired committee hearings on the proposed law at the state capital and at each of the state institutions. Because of the tremendous backlash against the efforts to close the state institutions, we knew the hearings would be packed with parents and employees of the institution opposed to closing institutions and in support of the proposed law.

The first hearing, held at the State Capitol in Harrisburg, was packed. Our most experienced leaders, who had been residents of institutions, signed up to testify, but they were not allowed to speak. Ray Gagne was the only person with disabilities who was allowed to testify and Representative Fairchild attacked him verbally. Prior to this, we had formed a partnership with the independent living centers and ADAPT activists were in attendance to support us at the hearings.

The ADAPT activists had extensive experience in power politics and we had none. Our leadership admired them. The ADAPT members attended in significant numbers and lined the walls of the room. They did not testify or speak but were there to give our leaders support and strength and to bear witness to the proceedings. They made a huge contribution to our efforts just by their presence.

The hearings were tumultuous and painful. Before each hearing, we would tour the institution and meet as many people as we could. It was hard to see so many people living in such isolation. It was difficult for all of us to stand up against such opposition, such animosity, but we knew we were speaking for the people still living there who yearned for the chance to live in the community. Carolyn Morgan, board president, used to tell everyone, "We just have to tap into our resources within ourselves. We can and we will make a difference."

The hearing at Polk State Center was the most difficult. Polk has long been considered one of the worst institutions in the state. It was located in the far northwestern region of Pennsylvania and hours from any major city. It was the major employer in the area. The Committee Hearing was held in the institution's auditorium. There were about three hundred parents and staff people present. The committee members sat up on a big stage. We had two people testify who used to live at Polk. As they gave their testimony, there was silence in the audience. No one could dispute the truth of the voices of the people who had actually lived there. We had placed a booklet we had published showing the success stories of people who had moved out of institutions on each of the three hundred seats in the auditorium. Not one copy was left behind after everyone had left the auditorium.

What turned out to be the last hearing was held at Woodhaven Center in Philadelphia on October 15, 1997. Woodhaven was an unusual institution of three hundred residents that was a state facility operated by the Temple University Institute for Disabilities. It was initially designed to be a model program for people with behavioral problems, but by the time it was built and operationalized its time had passed. Community programs were sprouting up and the benefits of community living were becoming abundantly clear. However, the Woodhaven institution persisted in attempting to be a "model program."

At the Woodhaven hearing, Representative Fairchild decreed that no person with disabilities would be allowed to testify. We planned a rally outside the hearing room to protest not being permitted to testify. We arranged for the leaders of the national self-advocacy organization, Self-Advocates Becoming Empowered, to attend. Tia Nelis, chairperson of the group and a strong leader from People First of Illinois, participated with us along with ADAPT and other advocates. Twelve cross-disability organizations became sponsors of the rally. Debbie Robinson served as the coordinator, and in a pre-rally press release the leaders of Speaking for Ourselves stated:

- "We are trying to get all the people out of the State institutions." —Steve Dorsey, vice president of Speaking for Ourselves.
- "It's a violation of the constitution to not let us speak." —Octavia Green, board president of Speaking for Ourselves.
- "These hearings have treated people with disabilities in a barbaric way. The Legislators think we are not human as if we don't have any brains." —Debbie Robinson, board member and organizer of the Campaign for Freedom Rally.

More than 150 people attended the rally, but toward the end of the hearing, people's anger boiled over at not being allowed to testify, and they shut down the proceedings. Through marching, singing, and megaphones, the people made their voices heard. That was the last hearing ever held. While the bill did pass the legislature, Governor Tom Ridge vetoed the measure.

In 1997, Debbie Robinson was appointed by President Clinton to serve on the National Council on Disabilities (NCD). Justin Dart had recommended her to the president for this very prestigious position. One day, an FBI agent appeared in the Speaking for Ourselves office and began asking questions about Debbie. He told us he was doing a background check. Unbeknownst to us, Debbie's appointment had to be approved by the United States Senate and required an

FBI character investigation. The FBI interviewed everyone, including Debbie's mother, family, friends, neighbors, and coworkers at her job.

Following Debbie's appointment to the NCD, she attended a special meeting on September 10, 1997, with President Clinton and Vice President Gore at the White House. Only twelve national disability leaders had been asked to meet directly with the president and Debbie was one of them. Walking into the White House to meet with the president was both inspiring and intimidating. The meeting was held in the historic Cabinet Room. Surprisingly, Debbie was seated in the chair next to the president. The other disability leaders kidded Debbie about sitting in what they called the "hot seat."

Debbie was given one minute to address the president. She was very nervous. Debbie spoke about how important the ADA was and said: "It gave us our civil rights and has improved transportation and jobs and more importantly given people the feeling like they have rights. We need your support, Mr. President." She finished by asking the president for his support in getting people with disabilities out of institutions and into the community. "Mr. President, you need to speak more about these issues. When you give talks on TV, you don't talk about disability issues. You need to bring this up more to the public. We need to hear your voice supporting us and the ADA." The president said, "You are right, I need to do more on that."

As part of Debbie's duties as an NCD member, she traveled to many states for hearings and council business. On one trip to Atlanta, Debbie and I were able to visit the Martin Luther King museum, where Debbie met and talked to Coretta Scott King, Dr. King's widow. Debbie's personal success story was later told in the book *Women with Intellectual Disabilities*[17] and in her oral history.

In 1999, our participation in SABE and its network of disability activists led to our first efforts to expand self-determination in Pennsylvania. The Robert Wood Johnson Foundation had funded a national effort to develop and fund self-determination. They were sponsoring conferences across the country in regions. Speaking for Ourselves served as the host for the Northeast Regional Conference. One thousand people attended from eleven states. It was the only self-determination conference planned and hosted by people with disabilities and remains the largest conference ever held on self-determination in the United States.

In 2000, Debbie Robinson organized the first Freedom March to the Pennsylvania capital in Harrisburg. We marched four blocks through the streets of Harrisburg and held the largest rally of the year under the Capitol Dome. More than three hundred people participated, representing more than twenty cross-disability organizations. People came from all over the state. The rally was covered in newspapers in Erie, Pittsburgh, Allentown, Harrisburg, and Philadelphia. The following year, SABE called for similar marches to be held all over the country on the same day.

It would have been impossible to imagine in 1981 that from the small beginning of five people meeting in an old run-down house that served as the headquarters of the local Arc, a self-advocacy movement would develop that would affect people across the country, or that former residents of Pennhurst would stand up, at first in local self-advocacy chapters and later at national conferences, and speak about the abuse and horror of institutions. No one present at those meetings would have envisioned that they and their fellow advocates would one day take their stories and message around the world, that in person, at conferences, and in books, their words and stories would inspire thousands of people to fight to "free the people" living in institutions.

Since that time, thirteen states have closed all their state institutions. Five more states are on the path to closing their state institutions in the next few years. Today, there are fewer than thirty thousand people with disabilities still living in state institutions—down from the 1968 high of over two hundred thousand. As Steve Dorsey, past Speaking for Ourselves board president, says, "We have to keep fighting to get everyone out into the community." The fight goes on.

## Postscript: "Close the Doors" (Self-Advocates Song)

***Chorus***
Close the doors
Close the doors

Close the doors
Behind us forever
Cus we deserve better
Til you throw away the key
I won't have my dignity
I won't be really free to live
While my brother's locked away
While my sister's in that place
I can't see the light of day myself
Til the day you can announce
That you've torn the last one down
You will hear me calling loud and
 clear
***Chorus***
Close the doors, close the doors,
 close the doors
Behind us forever
. . . Cuz we deserve better



## Notes

1. Halderman v. Pennhurst State School and Hospital, 446 F. Supp. 1295 (F.D. Pa. 1977).
2. *People First*, produced by James Stansfield (United States: James Stanfield Company, 1976), film.
3. Gunnar Dybwad and Hank Bersani, *New Voices: Self-Advocacy by People with Disabilities* (Cambridge, Mass.: Brookline Books, 1996).
4. Personal notes on Speaking for Ourselves, Mark M. Friedman.
5. Ruthie-Marie Beckwith, "The Bruises Are on the Inside: An Advisor's Perspective," in *Friendships and Community Connections Between People With and Without Developmental Disabilities*, ed. Angela Amado (Baltimore: Paul H. Brooks), 241–76.
6. Speaking for Ourselves. *Out of the Institution and You're Home Again: Success Stories, 1969–1999* (Pennsylvania: Speaking for Ourselves, 2000).
(Philadelphia: Speaking for Ourselves, 2000).
7. Mark M. Friedman and James W. Conroy, "Hiring Consumers to Interview Consumers About Day Program Satisfaction and Hopes: A Pilot Test," *Issues in Special Education and Rehabilitation* 5 (December 1988): 49–63.

8. Betty Potts, interviewed by Mark Friedman, Delaware County, Pennsylvania, October 10, 2013.

9. Karl Williams. "Held in Each Other's Hearts: Members of Speaking for Ourselves as told to Karl Williams," in *Friendships and Community Connections Between People With and Without Developmental Disabilities*, ed. Angela Amado (Baltimore: Paul H. Brooks, 1993), 241–76.

10. Radio interview with Roland Johnson, by Marty Moss-Coane, Philadelphia, WHYY, 1987.

11. *Out of the Institution and You're Home Again.*

12. Roland Johnson. *Lost in a Desert World: An Autobiography (as told to Karl Williams)* (Philadelphia: Speaking for Ourselves, Massey-Reyner, 1999).

13. Roland Johnson, interview by Mark Friedman, 1996; Steve Eidelman, interview by Lisa Sonneborn, "Growing Self-Advocacy Movement and Roland Johnson," in "Visionary Voices, " Temple University, Institute on Disability (2011).

14. On Justin Dart's life and legacy as a self-advocate, see Fred Fay and Fred Pelka, "Justin Dart: An Obituary (2002)" at http://www.disabilityhistory.org/people_dart.html#jdobit.

15. Debbie Robinson, interview by Lisa Sonneborn, "Visionary Voices," Temple University, Institute on Disabilities (2011). https://disabilities.temple.edu/voices/detailVideo.html?media=010-04.

16. Roland Johnson, "Who's in Control?" YouTube, http://www.youtube.com/watch?v=zFI7u6V_GvA.

17. Susan O'Connor, Ellen Fisher, and Debra Robinson, "Intersecting Cultures: Women of Color with Intellectual Disabilities," in *Women with Intellectual Disabilities: Finding a Place in the World*, ed. Kelley Johnson and Rannveig Traustadottir (Philadelphia: Jessica Kingsley, 2000), 229–39.

CHAPTER 8

# The Pennhurst Longitudinal Study and Public Policy

*How We Learned That People Were Better Off*

JAMES W. CONROY

The story of the Pennhurst Longitudinal Study is one of science, law, and public policy. What follows is an insider's view of how scientists, lawyers, and policymakers can interact in the real world. Through personal recollections woven with the findings of the study, it seeks to explore several themes. First, how did the first truly rigorous scientific study of deinstitutionalization of people with developmental and intellectual disabilities come about? Second, what did the study find out about the question "Are the people better off?" and how did it measure that? The findings surprised the study's principal investigator considerably. Third, did those findings stand up to the test of time and scientific replication? The findings of subsequent studies have been remarkably consistent across states and nations. Finally, in what ways did the study influence policy and practice in the United States—and elsewhere?

The first part of the story of the study inevitably includes the personal. I agreed to move from Washington, D.C., to Philadelphia to take a job at Temple University's new Developmental Disabilities Center in 1974. The Pennhurst lawsuit had just been filed in 1974 by attorney David Ferleger on behalf of Terri Lee Halderman and other people living at Pennhurst. Everyone working at the Temple Center knew that conditions at Pennhurst were appalling, because of Bill Baldini's 1968 Philadelphia television exposé. It appeared to us, the founders of the new academic center at Temple, that getting involved with this new lawsuit, as scientists, might be a good way to help make things better at Pennhurst and places like it.

By coincidence, I had some personal knowledge of the facility. In my first job out of college, in 1970, I worked on a national study of the impacts of a new federal law: the Developmental Disabilities Act of 1970. The consulting firm for which I worked had been contracted to determine the impacts of broadening the law from what was then called "mental retardation" to include people with cerebral palsy, epilepsy, and related conditions. Our primary method was to conduct a mail survey of the characteristics and needs of thousands of people receiving services and supports from preschools, schools, day programs, sheltered workshops, nursing homes, and specialized residential institutions.

Best survey science practice demanded that we check on the accuracy of what we were obtaining by mail. As the only member of the firm who had studied statistics in college, I was assigned to draw a representative sample of facilities to visit in person and check on ("validate") the data. We took all the national directories of facilities we could acquire and figured out a way to select a sample of fifty facilities such that every facility in the country had an equal probability of being selected—the definition of random sampling. The consulting firm's five research staff split up the random sample of facilities, ten each, and traveled to them in person. My assignment included a facility then called "Pennhurst State School and Hospital." In 1971, I drove from Washington to Spring City, Pennsylvania, and saw the conditions firsthand.

There I saw the unbelievable conditions first revealed by Bill Baldini's 1968 exposé *Suffer the Little Children*. For a young man with no prior experience of such things, the visit was life changing. I knew something had to be done, but did not know what.

By 1974, I had found work at Temple University in Philadelphia. Pennhurst was the hottest topic extant in Pennsylvania. Under the leadership of director Dr. Edward Newman, former commissioner of the U.S. Rehabilitation Services Administration, the new Temple University Developmental Disabilities Center (DDC) created a Legal Advocacy program. Meetings were arranged with Attorney Ferleger, and later with his colleagues at the Public Interest Law Center of Philadelphia. Our purpose was to find out how an academic center could assist in the mission of improving conditions at Pennhurst.

It became clear that a productive role for an academic center in such an unfolding legal and social policy battle would be to provide objective and scientific analysis of conditions and remedies—including gathering concrete evidence and providing highly qualified expert witnesses. The director and the staff of the fledgling Developmental Disabilities Center were unanimous in resolving to provide exactly that.[1]

Thus, as a very young man, I was able to get involved in the Pennhurst litigation in my official capacity as research coordinator of the DDC of Temple University. The first thing we needed, in my opinion, were hard facts about the qualities of life of, and services rendered to, the people at Pennhurst. At that time, there were about 1,240 people living there. I obtained a list via the attorneys and drew a "Simple Random Sample" of 124 people. Our request to the Court was for the complete "patient records" as they were then called for each person in the sample.[2]

These records provided much of the evidence that proved so telling in Court. For many months in 1976 and 1977, a team of research associates at Temple—including faculty, staff, and volunteers—analyzed the 124 records in successive "sweeps." We worked in a locked conference room at the Center. The attorneys visited regularly to see our progress and exchange legal thinking with social science thinking, all toward the goal of extracting the most telling evidence of quality and safety possible from the files.

In our first sweep, we pulled every instance of a person being seen by a psychologist or psychiatrist. We found that the average over the past decade had been three minutes per person per year. In a second sweep, we catalogued all habilitative programs and goals for each of the individuals. We noted that tooth-brushing programs were very common—about half the people were apparently being taught how to brush their teeth. One of my colleagues remarked on finding a person in a tooth-brushing program who had no teeth whatsoever. We swept through the 124 records a third time to count how many people actually had teeth. We learned that about a third of the people who were being taught to brush their teeth had no teeth.

Later, in court, we found that removing all teeth from people at Pennhurst had been commonplace for decades. It was a response to biting. People who bit others were, it was revealed, punished and programmed, but if the person bit again, the Pennhurst dentist would pull all teeth. The fact that even those people were often on tooth-brushing programs suggested that the so-called "habilitative programming" going on at Pennhurst might often be a sham.

Legally, two of the most important findings from the sampling study concerned loss of independent functioning skills and reports of abuse or neglect.

Because of prior review of rating scales of "adaptive behavior," which includes self-care, independent functioning, and functional abilities, I knew that the most commonly used measure over the preceding decades had been Edgar Doll's Vineland Social Maturity Scale.[3] The Vineland was a simple scale of 117 yes/no items ranging from basic abilities like "Stands Alone" and "Marks with Pencil or Crayon" up to higher-order skills like "Makes Telephone Calls" or "Assumes Responsibility Beyond Own Needs." Dr. Doll intended this scale as a more meaningful approach than the IQ, or Intelligence Quotient, for people with developmental and intellectual disabilities. The IQ emphasized academic skill, while the SQ—Social Quotient—emphasized functioning within our society.

We decided to find the earliest and the most recent Vineland scale for each of the 124 people in the sample. We could then see if people had gained or lost skills during their time at Pennhurst. By the time we did this analysis, the average person at Pennhurst had been there for twenty-four years. This gave us a fairly long time interval within which one or several Vineland scales might have been collected. It turned out that about half of our sample of 124 had two Vineland scales in their records.

What we found was that the average person in our sample had not gained in social maturity, or adaptive behavior, while living at

Pennhurst—in fact, the average person had regressed. Their Social Quotient scores had gone steadily down for every year they had been at Pennhurst.

This became crucial in court, because the sole Constitutional justification for taking away the freedom of a citizen—who had committed no crime—was to provide treatment that would *improve* their condition. The Vineland evidence showed that instead of providing benefit, living at Pennhurst had *caused harm.*

The 124-person records review also produced a great deal of evidence about abuse and neglect. Even though it was quite possible that most instances of abuse and neglect went unreported and undocumented, the records contained so much of this kind of material that it was nearly overwhelming—in both the evidentiary and the emotional senses.

When Judge Broderick handed down his decision in *Halderman v. Pennhurst* on December 23, 1977, we found that our evidence from the sample study had been effective. Judge Broderick wrote, "Testimony had revealed that Pennhurst provided such a dangerous, miserable environment for its residents that many of them actually suffered physical deterioration and intellectual regression during their stay at the institution."[4] In his order of March 17, 1978, the judge required that Pennsylvania create new homes and activities in the community for every person at Pennhurst.[5]

The Temple team under my direction immediately decided that society would need to know where people went, and whether their lives would get better or worse. Our guiding belief was that individual well-being was, or should be, the ultimate unit of accountability in social changes and innovations. To know this, we would need 1978 "baseline" information about their status—adaptive behavior, challenging behavior, health, safety, services, individual goals, and quality of life in general.

The key motivator for this decision developed during a 1977 trip by plaintiff attorneys, staff, and Temple experts to the Willowbrook Review Panel in Staten Island. Willowbrook was already notorious, because of Robert Kennedy's visits in the 1960s and Geraldo Rivera's coverage of the conditions there in the early 1970s.[6] In a meeting with key leaders of the Willowbrook panel, we learned that between 1972 and 1977, nearly two thousand people had moved out of Willowbrook. However, none of the Court's Review Panel officials knew where they had gone, or if they were "better off."

To me, this was completely unconscionable and unacceptable. I believed that making massive changes in the lives of thousands of vulnerable people absolutely demanded that we find out if those changes were good, bad, or indifferent. I resolved on that trip that the outcomes of the Pennhurst situation would be tracked and scientifically documented.

In 1978, the Temple University Developmental Disabilities Center Evaluation and Research Group convened a team of faculty, students, and volunteers to collect data on the characteristics, well-being, and services of all the people still living at Pennhurst. Without any formal funding, the Temple group obtained the necessary approvals and clearances and proceeded to fan out across the Pennhurst campus for about three weeks until we had completed a five-page survey form that we developed (the Behavior Development Survey) for every person living at Pennhurst on March 17, 1978.[7] There were 1,154 people living there on that date. The data we collected on that form formed the "baseline" upon which all future "pre- and post-" comparisons of developmental progress, individual goals, assessments of needs, and service delivery were based.

Soon after Judge Broderick's landmark decision in *Halderman v. Pennhurst*, the federal government agencies concluded that this was a decision of such policy import that it must be studied scientifically. Several elements of the federal executive branch were keenly interested in what Judge Broderick's decision might mean for policy, organization, funding, and service delivery. Sections of the Department of Health and Human Services began talks immediately, including the Rehabilitation Services Administration, the Administration on Developmental Disabilities, the Assistant Secretary for Planning and Evaluation, and what was then called the Health Care Financing Administration (now the Centers for Medicare and Medicaid Services). With rarely seen haste, the agencies devised an interagency funding scheme to support a longitudinal study of the impacts of the court order. A request for proposals was issued in late 1979, open for competitive bidding by research and policy-oriented organizations.

That request for proposals was issued in 1979 to conduct a "Pennhurst Longitudinal Study," and Temple University's Developmental Disabilities Center teamed up with the Temple Institute for Survey Research to assist with field data collection, and the Human Services Research Institute (HSRI) to perform policy analysis and comparative cost studies. The fact that Temple possessed baseline data for all the people at Pennhurst was likely a key factor in the victory.

The HSRI part of the Pennhurst study was concerned with history, policy, and costs. The initial history of the institution, the issue, and the lawsuit was a useful document, and it remains so today. The annual policy and implementation analyses proved valuable for local officials and advocates as well.[8]

The Temple part of the Pennhurst Longitudinal Study was focused on one simple question: "Are the people better off?" We wanted above all to find out where people went, into what kind of new homes and day programs and human relationships, and whether their lives had improved. To do this, we designed a study that included face-to-face visits and data collection with every person—1,154 people—every year, with multiple measures of quality of life and service, plus an annual family survey of every known next of kin.[9]

In the final analysis, the outcomes of any social change must be measured in terms of the qualities of life of the people affected. We believed that everything else was secondary to that simple and fundamental question.

## The Key Findings: "Are People Better Off?"

The following is a brief personal account of the findings of the Pennhurst study. The full methodology, instruments, and detailed findings are readily available online and in the published peer-reviewed literature. What follows here is a nontechnical, graphically oriented review of more than five years of intensive scientific work.[10]

In the interest of full disclosure of potential biases, it is proper for a modern scientist to make known his or her initial "hypotheses" about what he/she believed would be the most likely results of a study. My own initial bias was that the Pennhurst "experiment" of reintegrating residents into the community would fail. My opinion was based on the dismal record of "dumping" in the field of mental illness, in which state psychiatric hospitals began downsizing in 1955.

The national disgrace of our failure to fund community supports for people released from psychiatric hospitals was well known. I had done research in the mental health field for federal agencies in the early 1970s,[11] and so I knew that the Community Mental Health Act of 1963 had been passed by the Congress but had never been adequately funded. I had also read an article in *Scientific American*, a journal for which I had the utmost respect, that showed the magnitude of our national betrayal of people with mental illness.[12]

In fact, my first published article in a peer-reviewed journal was entitled "Trends In Deinstitutionalization of the Mentally Retarded,"[13] and it was written partly as a warning against deinstitutionalization of people with [what was then called] mental retardation. It also helped spur the development of a national tracking system on residential settings.[14]

Even today, the failure of early deinstitutionalization of citizens with mental illness is regarded as a national debacle. The Community Mental Health Act provided for community-based care as an alternative to institution-based services. Not all states agreed with the guidelines, fearing that state hospitals would be closed without adequate funding in place for community-based care. Once released, some patients would end up in group homes without the mental health supports they needed. This was particularly true in larger urban areas.

Between 1955 and 1980, a half-million Americans were discharged from mental hospitals. There are today more than three hundred thousand people with severe and chronic mental illness in jails and prisons, and approximately one hundred thousand nonelderly mental patients in nursing homes. Therapeutic treatment lags or is nonexistent in these settings. Compounding the problem, according to the most recent government statistics at least 40 percent of the nation's aggregate of a half-million chronically homeless report some form of mental health problem.[15]

It was in that context that I approached the task of evaluating the outcomes of Judge Broderick's order. Though it never mentioned "closure" of Pennhurst, the order did require community placement of everyone there—and I knew that the vast majority of the people there had very significant limitations and would not survive without extensive and well thought-out support systems. I expected that the Pennhurst Longitudinal Study's primary utility would be that it would provide "early detection" of massive problems, including mortality. Comparative mortality—institution and community—became a topic of intense contention later in the scientific, advocacy, and legal communities. The study's early detection would enable the Court and the Commonwealth to cease deinstitutionalization, or at least find ways to make it work.

The next section of this chapter shows how wrong I was.

In the Pennhurst Longitudinal Study, my team at Temple University's Developmental Disabilities Center studied the individual human effects of the district court's orders in *Halderman v. Pennhurst*. This order resulted in the transfer of all of the people living in a large state institution in Pennsylvania to small, supervised Community Living Arrangements (CLAs) in the communities from which they originally came. From 1979 to 1986, the Temple team visited every person every year and surveyed every next of kin or guardian about their opinions. There were 1,154 people in residence at Pennhurst on the date of Judge Raymond J. Broderick's historic order of March 17, 1978. My team immediately visited every one of those people and collected information about characteristics, abilities, behavior, health, and service needs. (Many of these people are *still* being tracked in monitoring systems that grew out of the Pennhurst study.) Every person was visited every year, and every family was sent a survey. We knew a tremendous amount about their quality of life over the period from 1978 to 1992. About half of the people did not use verbal language at all, and half were not fully continent regarding toilet needs. Table 8.1 shows that the Pennhurst people had very significant disabilities and challenges. Such people had never before been relocated from institution to community on such a large scale. Even with its pitfalls, this shift

TABLE 8.1 Characteristics of the people at Pennhurst in 1978.

| Characteristic | Average |
|---|---|
| Average age | 39 |
| Average years at Pennhurst | 24 |
| Percent male | 64% |
| Percent nonverbal | 50% |
| Percent with seizures | 33% |
| Percent not fully continent | 47% |
| Percent with aggressive behaviors | 40% |
| Percent labeled severe or profound | 85% |

to CLAs was a transformative, even revolutionary development in the disability rights campaign.

The three-person Community Living Arrangement was the prevailing program model in Pennsylvania at that time. These operated in regular houses or apartments. Each client had some degree of intellectual or developmental disability, and frequently they had multiple disabilities that had to be accommodated. Nearly all of the Pennhurst people went into homes with round-the-clock, twenty-four-hour staffing. The provider agencies were entirely private corporations, and of forty-three such agencies operating in the southeast region of Pennsylvania, all were nonprofit except one (founded in the 1930s).

### *Increased Independence (Adaptive Behavior)*

The graph below depicts the average increase in adaptive behavior over the course of the eight study years—that is, once people moved from institution to community. Adaptive behavior is a technical term for independent functioning—the ability to do the activities of daily living for oneself, rather than needing assistance. At the left of the graph is the average score of people when they were living at Pennhurst in 1978. Later, after hundreds of people moved out into community homes, their independence increased sharply—from 59.7 in 1978 to 70.8 in 1983.

As figure 8.1 shows, this increase in independence did not stop there. People continued to grow and learn and become more independent year after year following movement from institution to community. The more than five hundred people represented in the graph gained 9 percent in adaptive behavior upon community placement and then moved up to 12 percent by three years later and 14 percent at the last measurement in 1986.

Moreover, a matched comparison study (comparing each person who moved to a very similar person who stayed at Pennhurst—a so-called "twins study") showed that the adaptive behavior growth displayed by people who moved to CLAs was ten times greater than the growth displayed by matched people who remained at Pennhurst.[16]

In the time of these studies, the primary goal of services was to assist and allow people to reach their maximum level of independent functioning. The Pennhurst study's tracking of adaptive behavior showed, for the first time, that major gains were associated with community placement.

*Reduced Challenging Behavior*

Challenging behavior is a technical term for causing harm to self or others. We measured how often and how intensely such behaviors happened among the people who left Pennhurst. These behaviors included things like damaging property, running away, and physically hurting oneself. The improvements are shown on the graph titled "Improvements in Challenging Behavior." Again, the first few hundred people who moved out of Pennhurst showed improvement (less frequent and less severe challenging behaviors). This trend continued, with the first gain being about 1 percent, then 3 percent after three years in the community, and 6 percent by fourteen years after the original 1978 measurement.

Initially, in 1979, the families of the people at Pennhurst were very satisfied with the institution. They were also quite strongly opposed to community placement. At the beginning, 83 percent of families reported satisfaction with Pennhurst, and 72 percent opposed movement to the community.

We learned during the surveys that families strongly believed that their relatives needed medical care, and this was a very large component of their belief that the institutional setting was needed.

FIGURE 8.1 Adaptive behavior development, 1978–1986.

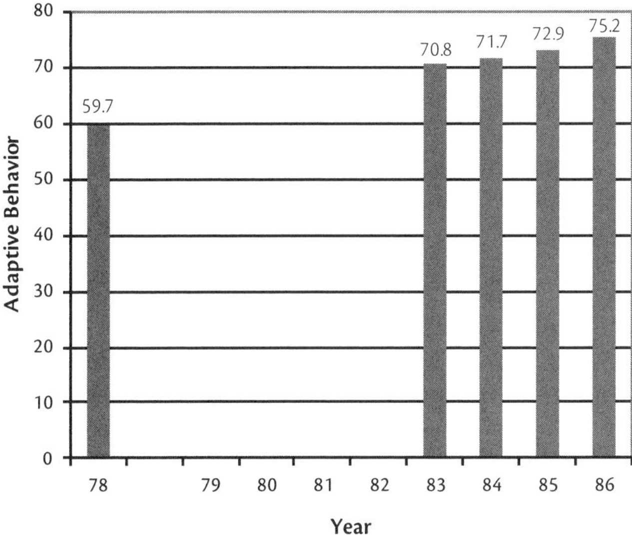


FIGURE 8.2 Improvements in challenging behavior.

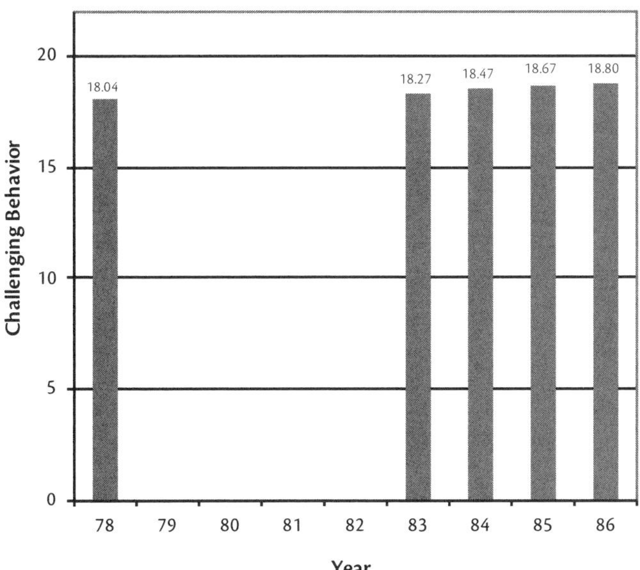

FIGURE 8.3 "Has your relative's general happiness changed since moving to the community?"

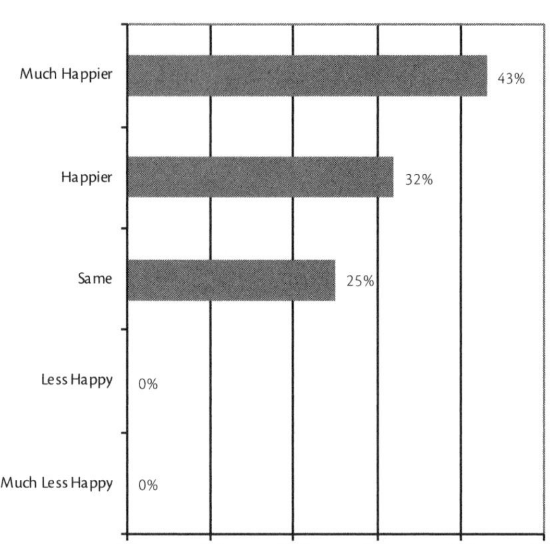


Via additional survey research, we linked this belief to the history of institutions that were created and marketed as "hospitals." We found that families perceived that their relatives had very intense needs for medical treatment, while day-to-day direct support workers did not have sufficient training to provide an adequate level of care.[17] When surveyed later, however, these families had radically changed their views. When asked whether they thought their relatives were happier or less happy since moving, not a single family rated their family member as being "less happy" or "much less happy." As shown in the 1991 survey results below, 75 percent of families thought their family member was happier. Not a single family believed their relative was less happy in the community. This and other related analyses showed that families had shifted in their feelings about community living, from strong opposition to overwhelming support.

Some of the most compelling findings in the study were the verbatim comments of the families after deinstitutionalization. These comments frequently included expressions of surprise that they (the parents) had ever opposed community placement in the first place, coupled with surprise at the magnitude of improvements in the qualities of their loved ones' lives.

*The Voices of the People Themselves—Happier, Never Go Back*

A crucial aspect of the Pennhurst study included "before and after" interviews with a random sample of fifty-six people from among those who were able to communicate—verbally or by other means. This aspect of the study was innovative. Prior to this study, researchers had apparently not felt that the feelings of the people themselves were worth investigating, or that they could not answer reliably enough.

After the move to the community, the proportion of people reporting satisfaction with various aspects of life was approximately double what was found in the institution. There were no areas of decreased satisfaction over the entire course of the study.[18] During fourteen years of tracking the people (we kept following all the people even after the longitudinal study ended), we noted only two people who said they would like to "go back." They were people who formerly had "the run of the place," in a sense similar to a trustee in a prison. They enjoyed great power and freedom within the institution.

Prior to Pennhurst closing in 1987, we tracked every public dollar expended to support a large sample of what we called "twins" at Pennhurst and in the community. Each "twin" at Pennhurst was matched with a "twin" who had already moved to the community—and who had the same gender, age, ethnicity, and general level of disability. In 1984 and thereafter, we published these studies in peer-reviewed scientific journals.[19]

The total public cost of serving the people who moved out of Pennhurst to Community Living Arrangements was significantly less than for the matched people still at Pennhurst—about $47,000 per year for people at Pennhurst, versus $40,000 for people in community living. However, the state had to pay a lot more for people in the community. These findings are illustrated in figure 8.4. Because federal funds were being used to help pay for Pennhurst, but not for community homes, Pennsylvania contributed only about $21,000 per year for people at Pennhurst, and about $36,000 per year for people in CLAs. Today, federal funds are readily available in community homes

FIGURE 8.4 Who pays? Federal, state, and local share of costs—institution versus community.

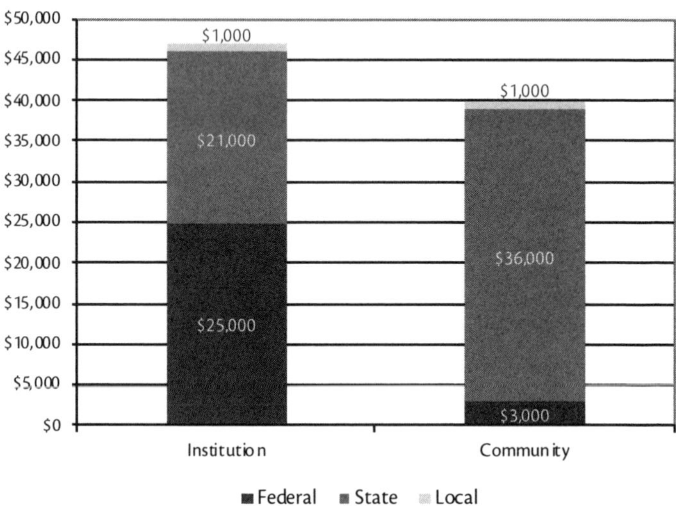


(via the Medicaid Home and Community Based Services program, commonly called Medicaid Waivers), so this "disincentive" for state governments to community living is gone.

The community settings did cost less than Pennhurst—but it is absolutely crucial to understand why. The entire cost savings could be traced to much lower salaries and benefits for community workers.[20] Pennhurst was staffed by state employees, and their powerful union had negotiated decent living wages over the decades. The community was new, not unionized, and direct support workers were paid close to minimum wage, often with no benefits. This situation persists today, and is widely believed to have significant consequences for quality, including high staff turnover, and the need for workers to hold two jobs.

The five years of the Pennhurst study led to the conclusion that, on the average, the people deinstitutionalized under the Pennhurst court order were better off in almost every way we knew how to measure. For the people who moved from Pennhurst to small community residences, results were conclusive. The study included ways of looking

TABLE 8.2 Pennhurst longitudinal study—summary of outcomes.

| | |
|---|---|
| Health | Access to health care was maintained; no deterioration of health or health care. |
| Qualities of environments | Major increases in measures of physical quality, individualization, and normalization. |
| Productivity | Increased: Daily engagement, activity, employment, earnings, household chores. From about 30 percent with daily program activities to nearly 100 percent. |
| Service delivery process | Increased services, from 189 to 225 hours per month; more teaching/training, therapies, goal attainment, case manager contact. |
| Integration | People "getting out" into places where they might encounter everyday citizens increased markedly. Family contacts were maintained. |

at quality of life beyond the ones highlighted above (increased independence, reduced challenging behavior, extremely positive reactions of relatives, and reduced public costs)—and these other measures of quality are summarized in table 8.2.

## The Consistency of the Conclusions

The Pennhurst research led me to try to replicate the study in other states, with and without court involvement. Replication is at the heart of science. I wanted to know whether the Pennhurst success could occur in other, different states and service systems.

While Pennhurst was being downsized, the state of New Hampshire determined to close its only institution, the Laconia State School. My colleagues and I completed the New Hampshire Applied Research Project in 1986. Our findings were precisely parallel to those we had obtained in the Pennhurst study.[21] Partly because of the positive findings of the New Hampshire study, community placement continued, and in 1991 New Hampshire became the first state to eliminate public institutionalization for people with intellectual and developmental disabilities.

TABLE 8.3 Comparative deinstitutionalization studies.

| State | Court-ordered? | Number of people | Number of years | Community model | Average age | % Severe/ profound | % Nonamb-ulatory | Years |
|---|---|---|---|---|---|---|---|---|
| PA | Yes | 1154 | 14 | 3 person | 43 | 86% | 18% | 78–92 |
| NH | Yes | 600 | 3 | 4 to 6 | 39 | 66% | 21% | 79–86 |
| LA | Yes | 268 | 5 | Varied | 25 | 68% | 17% | 80–86 |
| OK | Yes | 900 | 9 | Supp Liv | 25 | 86% | 27% | 90–99 |
| CT | Yes | 590 | 5 | Varied | 44 | 86% | 23% | 85–90 |
| CA | Yes | 2400 | 4 | 4 to 6 | 37 | 68% | 28% | 94–99 |
| NC | Yes | 900 | 4 | 4 to 6 | 46 | 26% | 12% | 92–99 |
| KS | No | 88 | 2 | 2 to 4 | 43 | 100% | 58% | 97–99 |
| IN | No | 200 | 1 | Supp Liv | 39 | 67% | 23% | 98–99 |
| NJ | No | 57 | 2 | 4 to 6 | 36 | 7% | 13% | 89–93 |
| Total | | 7157 | | | | | | |

Connecticut followed suit with its agreement to close the Mansfield Training School near Hartford, which was accomplished in 1993. The results were strikingly similar to both the Pennsylvania and the New Hampshire findings.[22]

During the ensuing two decades, the Center for Outcome Analysis has been involved in many of the major downsizing and closure efforts in the United States. We designed and operated the Gary W. Monitoring System in Louisiana, the Quality Assurance Project in Oklahoma, the Thomas S. Longitudinal Study in North Carolina, the Winfield Closure Study in Kansas, the Quality Tracking Project on Institutional Closures in Indiana, and the Quality Tracking Project related to the *Coffelt* settlement in California. The following table summarizes the major studies of deinstitutionalization by my team at the Center for Outcome Analysis.

The results of all these studies were extremely consistent. People in all of these deinstitutionalization efforts, in entirely different states and service systems, all gained in adaptive behavior (independent function or self-care abilities), became more capable of self-control (decreased behaviors that might harm self or others), became more integrated among nonhandicapped citizens, maintained their health, received more services, were treated far more as individuals and less as "one size fits all" groups, increased in the opportunity to make choices about their own lives, and they lived longer by far than they would have been expected to had they continued to live in an institution.[23]

After the Pennhurst study, a series of reports appeared in American scientific journals. There have been several literature review articles since then as well. One of the first reviews examined all published reports about behavioral gains and benefits of deinstitutionalization.[24] That review included several of our studies, and all were consistent in finding benefits similar to what we had reported in the Pennhurst study. More than a decade later, this review was repeated with identical results.[25] The behavioral outcomes, in terms of growth in self-care skills and independent functioning abilities, seem to be robust and have been widely replicated. The third decennial review was published in 2011,[26] confirming all prior summary conclusions.

The findings of the Pennhurst family surveys have also been subjected to a review for replication studies, and the results of that review fully supported the findings of the Pennhurst study.[27]

A recent thorough review of worldwide scientific literature on deinstitutionalization was performed by the Institute for Family Advocacy and Leadership Development of New South Wales, Australia, in 2007. They reviewed more than one hundred studies from nearly fifty years of research literature. In their executive summary, they concluded: "The evidence provides two important lessons for government. Firstly, that people with disability have better lives, measured in a myriad of ways, when they move out of institutions. Secondly, that whilst most families oppose the move to close institutions (change is always hard), families change their mind about its benefits after the move and become more and more committed to community living as time goes by."[28]

Even more recently, Raymond Lemay of Ontario, Canada, performed a review, in which he concluded, "People, irrespective of their degree of disability, are apt to do better in the community on most measures and do no worse when it comes to challenging behaviours. . . . Very simply, the institution cannot replace the community in providing individuals—including those with developmental and serious psychiatric disabilities—with the opportunities for the good life. There are no compelling client-related arguments left for keeping people with cognitive limitations, and possibly people with psychiatric disabilities, away from their families and communities."[29]

To my knowledge, every study that has thus far been performed has confirmed the simple conclusion of the Pennhurst Longitudinal Study: people who move from institutional to community living are, on the average, far "better off."

*The Specter of Community Mortality—Discredited Studies Still Being Cited*

Over the past twenty years, there has been one issue that temporarily questioned the success of deinstitutionalization in the field of intellectual and developmental disabilities. The issue of survival (mortality) merits close review. During Pennhurst, an organization of pro-institutional parents and members of institutional employee unions banded together to oppose the policy of deinstitutionalization. The group, the Voice of the Retarded, is still active at the time of this writing (see https://www.vor.net). Attorneys and scientists recruited by the Voice of the Retarded to support their pro-institutional viewpoint have appeared at every court case about institutions since Pennhurst.

In 1996, a study done in California concluded that the risk of dying was 72 percent higher in community group homes than in state institutions.[30] (They also found deaths to be 72 percent higher for people living with their own parents than for people living in public institutions. This was extremely difficult to find credible, and raised my suspicions right away.) It was based on a complex mathematical "model" of mortality. The data were provided to the two researchers by the California Department of Developmental Services and the California Department of Vital Statistics. This study was followed by several others, published in several journals. Each one was based on the original data from California.

It should be noted that David Strauss and Theodore Kastner received significant long term research support from the Voice of the Retarded, an organization explicitly founded to halt the movement from institution to community.

These studies have been brought to each and every court case and legislative deliberation concerning deinstitutionalization in the United States since 1996, including a joint legislative hearing in New Jersey in May of 2013.[31]

The studies were indeed frightening at first. I too was alarmed, and contacted the researchers directly to exchange ideas and follow-up studies. I asked one question, which Kastner emphatically denied: "Were any terminally ill people in the institutions moved to Intensive Care Units in community hospitals—and did they die there—and were they counted as 'community deaths' in your study?"

Today, the scientific community knows well that this is exactly what Strauss and Kastner did. They counted institutional deaths incorrectly. Many of the deaths they counted as "community deaths" were actually people who, dying at a state institution, were moved to local hospitals for intensive care at the end of their lives and died in those hospitals. Strauss, Kastner, and all their publication colleagues who followed counted them as "community deaths." They then based all their subsequent analyses, regression models, conclusions, and publications on simple miscounts.

This was demonstrated conclusively by Dr. K. Charlie Lakin of the University of Minnesota's Residential Information Systems Project in 1999.[32] As the head of the Residential Information Systems Project, Dr. Lakin had been receiving reports of deaths in all of America's public institutions from the California Department of Developmental Services (DDS) since the early 1980s. His data were so different from those used by Strauss and Kastner that he double checked them with another source, the Association of Public Developmental Disabilities Administrators (APDDA), which was comprised of the directors of all the public institutions. The APDDA also kept data on the population of people in institutions in every state, including deaths. The APDDA source agreed with Lakin's direct reports from the California Department of Developmental Services (DDS) within eight deaths: DDS 534, APDDA 526.

Lakin calculated from the Strauss and Kastner publications that they had counted between 352 and 418 deaths of people at California's institutions in their study. Thus they had counted 149 (plus or

TABLE 8.4 Reported and estimated deaths in California's institutions from fiscal years 1985 to 1994.

| California and national database reports | Number used by Strauss, Kastner, and colleagues |
|---|---|
| Between 526 and 534 | Between 352 and 418 |

minus 33) *fewer* deaths among California's institutional residents than were reported by the state's institutional superintendents *or* the national association of superintendents. (Lakin could not compute precise numbers from Strauss and Kastner's publications, and they refused to share any data in any way with Lakin's team, including Dr. Mary Hayden, so he had to estimate the range from their numbers.) Table 8.4 relates the simple tale as told by the numbers.

Thus the entire body of work about mortality in California's institutional versus community settings was founded on simple miscounting. They miscounted more than one hundred deaths out of about 352 to 534—somewhere between a fifth and a third of all the deaths has been misclassified. This easily accounts for their erroneous conclusion that the probability of mortality was 72 percent higher in community residential settings than in state institutions.

The Strauss and Kastner mortality findings have never been replicated here or in any other country. Replication is the ultimate criterion for scientific credibility. All subsequent studies have failed to confirm or support the Strauss and Kastner work.[33] Moreover, the one study based on the actual experience of the Pennhurst people found that people tended to live *longer* in the community than they would have if they had remained in an institution.

The Pennhurst Longitudinal Study had a tremendous impact on policy. As soon as results began to appear in the early 1980s, Pennsylvania officials were encouraged to continue the movement of people from Pennhurst into the community. Judge Broderick cited the results in his later rulings and opinions, including the final settlement agreement, to justify his decision. The attorneys who argued to end institutional models "took their show on the road." The Public Interest Law Center of Philadelphia (PILCOP) obtained a large grant from the U.S. Administration on Developmental Disabilities to offer workshops around the country, teaching other advocacy attorneys how to mount a similar lawsuit in their own states. And, indeed, lawsuits were initiated in at least ten other states, specifically modeled after the *Halderman v. Pennhurst* case. PILCOP attorneys assisted in many of those lawsuits.

As those lawsuits proceeded in other states, I was called in as an expert witness (subpoenaed, and without pay) in many of them. I described the extremely positive findings of the Pennhurst Longitudinal Study, and that allowed judges to feel some confidence that people would be better off if they moved from institution to community.

I was called to testify before the U.S. Senate committee concerned with amending the Medicaid statute too because of its "inherent institutional bias."[34] I found that several of the committee members were surprised at the positive outcomes of the Pennhurst closure, because they too were familiar with the nation's dismal record of deinstitutionalization in the mental health field.

At the time of this writing, fourteen states have closed all of their public institutions for people with intellectual and developmental disabilities. None have reported plans to return to the old model. It is now taken as established public policy knowledge that no one "needs" to live in a large, isolated, segregated institutional setting.

The influence of the study has extended internationally, as well. In 2006, New Zealand became the first entire nation to end public institutions entirely. By a great coincidence, the man who helped involve Bill Baldini in the 1968 exposé was instrumental in making this "first" nationwide closure happen. Ed Goldman, who worked for the Arc of Philadelphia in 1968, later became Pennsylvania's first Commissioner of Mental Retardation (now called Deputy Secretary of the Office of Developmental Programs) and helped implement the Right to Education, and later the creation of the community living system. From 1986 to 1993, he worked in New Zealand's service system and, in that role, oversaw the move of hundreds of people from institutional to community settings. He cited the Pennhurst study and overcame bureaucratic reluctance and much of the family fears by using scientific evidence that the change would be beneficial.

The Pennhurst study, and all the studies modeled after it, have been the subject of seminars, workshops, lectures, classes, presentations, and speeches all over the world. Venues have included the Duma in Moscow, the Ministry of Finance in Lithuania, Haifa University in Israel, the association of institutional directors in Serbia, the fledgling association of self-advocates named Ne Per Ne in Kosovo, a cross-country lecture tour of Mexico in 2011, the 2011 annual conference of attorneys working with various initiatives of the Open Society Foundation in Ireland, a 2012 gathering of all national disability group representatives in the Republic of Georgia, and a gathering of disability organization representatives in Ukraine in 2014. There have been many others.

In the concluding portion of this volume, we will discuss the passage and early impacts of the United Nations Convention on the Rights of Persons with Disabilities. Article 19 establishes "the equal right of all persons with disabilities to live in the community." The world is changing now. The significance of Pennhurst, and the Pennhurst Longitudinal Study, is that it is the evidence-based realization that there is a "better way" to support people with disabilities—better than the outmoded and inevitably pernicious model of large-scale segregation, isolation, and abuse.

## Notes

1. University officials were "not so sure" that we should assist in a lawsuit against the Commonwealth. Temple University was a quasi–state institution itself, with major Commonwealth funding. However, claims of academic freedom and the fact that our funding was primarily federal were the arguments that prevailed.

2. How those records were obtained is a tale not to be omitted. The Court asked the Department of Justice for help in this process of "discovery" of evidence. The Department of Justice includes the Federal Bureau of Investigation. Unbeknownst to us at the time, agents of the FBI appeared unannounced at Pennhurst with full legal warrant authority, and obtained access to the files of the 124 people. The agents then proceeded to photograph every page of every person's file. Some people had one thousand pages accumulated over forty or more years at Pennhurst. The film was taken back to Washington, developed into 8 × 12 photos, and then these photos were copied onto paper, sheet by sheet. A set of 124 exact duplicates of the patient records was ultimately delivered to Temple University by officers of the Court. The cost must have been staggering.

3. Edgar A. Doll, "Preliminary Standardization of the Vineland Social Maturity Scale," *American Journal of Orthopsychiatry* 6, no. 2 (1936): 283–93.

4. Halderman v. Pennhurst State School and Hospital, 446 F. Supp. 1295 (E.D. Pa. 1977) at 1308 and 1318.

5. Judge Broderick issued both a decision (December 23, 1977) and an order (March 17, 1978). The decision asked the parties to come to a compromise—a settlement agreement. They could not. Hence the judge was forced to issue an order, which gave Pennsylvania no choices and no room for negotiation. It was the first order in this area of litigation—all prior actions about institutional conditions had ended in settlements.

6. Mr. Rivera obtained the idea of covering Willowbrook via the dissemination of the Bill Baldini 1968 exposé of Pennhurst. Baldini's station and network sent out dozens of copies of the film, and recommended that local affiliates replicate what Mr. Baldini had done. Although Rivera's work garnered far more national recognition than Baldini's, it was not the pioneering effort.

7. March 17, 1978, was the date of Judge Raymond Broderick's order for community placement.

8. The HSRI final report, however, was deemed unacceptable in December 1985 by the HHS project officer, and required thorough rewriting by the Temple principal investigator over the December holiday break while the HSRI principal was on vacation. Moreover, the HSRI cost comparisons unfortunately never produced clear or publishable conclusions, and the Temple team took the lead on this aspect as well, with several studies and journal publications (e.g., Jones, Conroy, Feinstein, and Lemanowicz, 1984).

9. Two great advantages of the "every person every year" approach were: (1) sampling was not used, so inferential statistical tests were not strictly even necessary—they are intended for generalizing from a sample to a larger population. We had the entire population. (2) The credibility factor—when nonscientists heard the phrase, "We have visited every person every year," the impact upon trust in the findings was powerful. James W. Conroy and Valerie J. Bradley, "The Pennhurst Longitudinal Study: Combined Report of Five Years of Research and Analysis," Office of the Assistant Secretary for Planning and Evaluation Report, March 1, 1985, https://aspe.hhs.gov/basic-report/pennhurst-longitudinal-study-combined-report-five-years-research-and-analysis.

10. Ibid.

11. Joel Levy, Edward Newman, and James W. Conroy, *Models for Program Improvement: Alternative Approaches to Planning for Mental Health Services* (Washington, D.C.: LMC Inc., 1974).

12. Ellen L. Bassuk and Samuel Gerson, "Deinstitutionalization and Mental Health Services," *Scientific American* 238 (1989): 46–53.

13. James W. Conroy, "Trends in Deinstitutionalization of the Mentally Retarded," *Mental Retardation* 15 (1977): 44–46.

14. K. Charlie Lakin, personal communication with James W. Conroy, 1994.

15. "Homelessness Statistics by State," https://www.usich.gov/tools-for-action/map; "The State of Homelessness in America," https://endhomelessness.org/homelessness

-in-america/homelessness-statistics/state-of-homelessness-report-legacy. The National Alliance to End Homelessness mirrors government statistics, citing a total of 553,000 homeless in 2018.

16. James W. Conroy and Valerie Bradley, *The Pennhurst Longitudinal Study: A Report of Five Years of Research and Analysis* (Philadelphia: Temple University Developmental Disabilities Center; Boston: Human Services Research Institute, 1985).

17. James W. Conroy, Celia S. Feinstein, James A. Lemanowicz, and Mersina Kopatsis, "Medical Needs of Institutionalized Mentally Retarded Persons: Perceptions of Families and Staff Members," *American Journal of Mental Deficiency* 89 (1985): 510–14.

18. James W. Conroy, Robert Walsh, and Celia S. Feinstein, "Consumer Satisfaction: People with Mental Retardation Moving from Institutions to the Community," vol. 3, 135–50, of *Advances in Mental Retardation and Developmental Disabilities*, ed. Steven Breuning and Robert Gable (Greenwich, Conn.: JAI Press, 1987).

19. Philip Jones, James W. Conroy, Celia S. Feinstein, and James A. Lemanowicz. "A Matched Comparison Study of Cost Effectiveness: Institutionalized and Deinstitutionalized People," *Journal of the Association for Persons with Severe Handicaps* 9 (1984): 304–13.

20. Roger J. Stancliffe and K. Charlie Lakin. "Costs and Outcomes of Community Services for Persons with Intellectual and Developmental Disabilities," *Research and Training Center on Community Living Policy Research Brief* 14, no. 1 (2004).

21. Valerie Bradley, James W. Conroy, Susan Covert, and Celia Feinstein. *Community options: The New Hampshire Choice* (Cambridge, Mass.: Human Services Research Institute, 1986).

22. James W. Conroy, James A. Lemanowicz, Celia S. Feinstein, and Joan Bernotsky. *1990 Results of the CARC v. Thorne Longitudinal Study: The Connecticut Applied Research Project* (Havertown, Pa.: Center for Outcome Analysis, 1991).

23. James W. Conroy and Miriam Adler, "Mortality Among Pennhurst Class Members, 1978 to 1989: A Brief Report," *Mental Retardation* 36, no. 5 (1998): 380–85.

24. Sheryl A. Larson and K. Charlie Lakin, "Deinstitutionalization of Persons with Mental Retardation: Behavioral Outcomes," *Journal of the Association for Persons with Severe Handicaps* 14 (1989): 324–32.

25. Shannon Kim, Sheryl A. Larson, and K. Charlie Lakin, "Behavioral Outcomes of Deinstitutionalization for People with Intellectual Disability: A Review of U.S. Studies Conducted Between 1980 and 1999," *Journal of Intellectual and Developmental Disabilities* 26, no. 1 (2001): 15–34.

26. K. Charlie Lakin, Sheryl A. Larson, and Shannon Kim, "Behavioral Outcomes of Deinstitutionalization for People with Intellectual and/or Developmental Disabilities: Third Decennial Review of U.S. Studies, 1977–2010," *Policy Research Brief, Research and Training Center on Community Living, University of Minnesota* 21, no. 2 (2011): 1–11.

27. Sheryl A. Larson and K. Charlie Lakin, "Parent Attitudes About Residential Placement Before and After Deinstitutionalization: A Research Synthesis," *Journal of the Association for Persons with Severe Handicaps* 16 (1991): 25–38.

28. IFALD (Institute for Family Advocacy and Leadership Development), "Presenting the Evidence—Deinstitutionalization: A Review of the Literature," New South Wales, Australia, 2007, https://scholarworks.wmich.edu/jssw/vol9/iss4/7.

29. Raymond A. Lemay, "Deinstitutionalization of People With Developmental Disabilities: A Review of the Literature," *Canadian Journal of Community Mental Health* 28, no. 1 (2009).

30. David Strauss and Theodore Kastner, "Comparative Mortality of People with Mental Retardation," *American Journal on Mental Retardation* 101 (1996): 26–40.

31. Andrew Kitchenman, "Families of Disabled Residents Sue to Keep Developmental Centers Open," *NJ Spotlight* (newsletter), June 6, 2013, https://www.njspotlight.com/stories/13/06/05/families-of-disabled-residents-sue-to-keep-developmental-centers-open.

32. K. Charlie Lakin, "Observations on the California Mortality Studies," *Mental Retardation* 36 (1999): 395–400.

33. Kevin F. O'Brien and E. S. Zaharia, "Recent Mortality Patterns in California," *Mental Retardation* 36 (1998): 372–79; Paul Lerman, Dawn Apgar, and Tameeka Jordan, "Deinstitutionalization and Mortality: Findings of a Controlled Research Design in New Jersey," *Mental Retardation* 41, no. 4 (2003): 225–36; Kelly Hsieh, Tamar Heller, and Sally Freels, "Residential Characteristics, Social Factors, and Mortality Among Adults with Intellectual Disabilities: Transitions out of Nursing Homes," *Intellectual and Developmental Disabilities* 47, no. 6 (2009): 447–65.

34. James W. Conroy, *Results of the Pennhurst Longitudinal Study*, Washington, D.C.: Testimony presented to the United States Senate, Committee on Finance, Subcommittee on Health, September 1986.

## PART 3

# A View to the Future

In the years following its 1987 closing, the Pennhurst campus became both a site of conscience and a site for paranormal-seeking urban adventurers. As such its presence and current condition raise questions about historic preservation and purposeful reuse. Part 3 includes chapters that explore site conditions and possible new uses for the sprawling compound of now vacant building and grounds. Even as advocates demanded a dignified and socially constructive preservation, the Pennhurst Asylum, a macabre fright-night commercial venture, has flourished. Equally disturbing is the willingness of successive property owners to dismantle the original structures in the hopes of selling off large parcels, a process that is now underway. These tendencies raise fundamental questions bearing on hundreds of similar institutions that lay dormant and in ruin. What do you do with these extensive holdings that have been idled and in disrepair for decades? How does society memorialize the sites of atrocity and failed public policy in an age of commercial development?

CHAPTER 9

# Touring the Ecology of the Abandoned

HEATH HOFMEISTER AND CHRIS PEECHO CADWALADER

Between 1992 and 2008, Pennhurst served as both a sign and a symbol of what could befall public institutions that have closed in the United States—more than two hundred in all. At Pennhurst, the story involved official government neglect, and a few weak rumblings about historic preservation. After the dawn of the new millennium, there was a surge of underground explorers, including simultaneous elements of reverence, interest in the paranormal, and destructive impulses. The era of thrill-seeking "urban exploration" (1992–2008) yielded to the sale of the property to commercial developers, who, among other money-making schemes, incorporated a Halloween fright-night attraction on the grounds in 2010.

For eighty years a human tide had steadily flowed into the wide doors of Pennhurst's numerous halls, trapping victims caught in the legal and societal push of those lawfully sanctioned currents. Outrage, advocacy, and legal action changed that, and Pennhurst saw its last residents leave and the doors padlocked in the fall of 1987. Appropriately, great attention was paid to the future of the people who lived at Pennhurst; a definitive plan was set in place for those individuals to move forward into greatly improved circumstances. In contrast, for thirty years after the last resident departed, little or no planning was done for the physical complex.

State institutions across the country vary in how they have reused, modified, or demolished structures, but at Pennhurst there has been a short-lived interest in historic preservation. Unfortunately, the motivations of private ownership led to a stunningly disrespectful use of the property. Today, these commercial interests coexist with the desire for efforts at dignified remembrance of what happened at Pennhurst and places like it.

## Decades of Neglect and Decay

So rapid, unplanned, and complete was the evacuation of Pennhurst after its official closure that much was left as it had been on the campus: paperwork left on desks, beds sitting in wards, and toothbrushes at sinks in empty residence halls. File cabinets, records, and a great deal of confidential material was left in the wake of the final exodus. Volumes were discarded or transferred to mold-infested cellars at Norristown State Hospital or other sites. Some materials did make it to the State Archives in Harrisburg. The imposing edifices remained standing and idled for decades. Once discarded, these physical artifacts became "finds" for the waves of urban explorers that discovered and made the campus a destination for discovery.

For more than two decades, Pennhurst State School was an abandoned city, literally suspended in time as residential and commercial development encroached on the property. The Commonwealth of Pennsylvania simply turned out the lights, locked the doors, and drove away, leaving the buildings to weather the ravages of time and the elements on their own. Patient files were left behind, with little thought of confidentiality, and the potential for souvenir hunters to wander the grounds increased over the years.

Horizon Hall and several of the new buildings dating from the 1960s "New Pennhurst" program were ceded to the Commonwealth of Pennsylvania's Department of Military Affairs for use as the Southeastern Veterans Center.[1] A retirement facility and medical clinic stand on the site today. The former Female Colony, also known as Pennhurst's "upper campus," was transferred to the Pennsylvania National Guard for administrative offices and an armory.

Another part of "The Plan" called for all of the functional furnishings and equipment to be transported to Capitol Hall on the upper campus, where they were warehoused. This cache was made available to other state schools and hospitals (like Whitehaven, South Mountain, and Polk), as they had need for such resources. In this way Pennhurst Center, as the complex was called in its final phase, was opened to other state institutions for harvesting needed resources. Beds, equipment, and even room partitions were pulled from Pennhurst for use in other facilities.

Amazingly, just as Pennhurst was closing, some long overdue maintenance projects were just being completed. For example, the auditorium was brought up to ADA compliance (Americans with Disabilities Act) shortly before the doors were padlocked.

For a number of years, the security personnel from the Department of Military Affairs, who were once employed at Pennhurst, continued to patrol the shuddered lower campus. This practice was discontinued when the closed property became popular with "unofficial" visitors, and managing the campus became more hazardous.

The largest factor in the "abandonment" of the Pennhurst complex was budgetary. As the buildings and grounds were no longer needed, little money was allocated for upkeep. A large part of this dynamic is found in the way that state and federal resources are managed. In Pennsylvania, as in other states, the facilities, grounds, and resources are owned and maintained by the state General Services Administration (GSA). State agencies, like the Pennsylvania Department of Public Welfare, will "rent" facilities from the state GSA out of their operating budgets. This was the case with Pennhurst Center; the Department of Welfare ran the programs and services provided at Pennhurst, while the state GSA ran the buildings. When Pennhurst was no longer needed, the GSA no longer budgeted money to maintain the facilities, and the buildings and grounds fell into rapid decline.

As seasons passed, heat and frost worked to chip the masonry façades and curl the lead paint from the walls. The once carefully manicured grounds were left to grow wild, saplings rising from the lawns and standing trees growing thick and crowding the buildings. Roofs that had leaked on residents in years prior continued to leak, while seasons and the elements worked to loosen and penetrate those slate roofs that had previously been water tight. Leaves clogged rain gutters and storm drains. Water dripped through ceilings and floors and collected in basements and tunnel systems.

Past the turn of the century, the historic Pennhurst campus remained a silent and decaying city. Residents of the adjacent Spring City neighborhoods walked the ring of Commonwealth Drive and admired the changing seasons against the backdrop of the grand, aging buildings. As the years passed, local knowledge of the campus's purpose and identity began to fade. After a decade, Pennhurst State School was not forgotten but was certainly less vividly known—a place visited only by locals and the intrepidly curious.

Just as the structure of Pennhurst was made physically vulnerable through abandonment by the Commonwealth, the symbolic meaning of Pennhurst was left to uncertain ends. The closure of the state school complex was a great testimony to the human desire for freedom and a collective effort for justice. However, without a firm reminder of the phenomenon of the civil rights struggle that occurred at Pennhurst, the meaning of the place and its history rapidly began to yield to neglect and decay. In losing its known identity, the campus silently shifted from being a cradle of liberation to a site devoid of known meaning, a stark and haunting oddity that stood ripe for projected meaning. The historical symbol of human triumph that was Pennhurst State School was lost to the fog of public ignorance, free to be exploited through misunderstanding and cruel, gothic imaginings.

## Urban Exploration: Dualism and the Assignment of New Meanings

While the historical purpose and meaning of the Pennhurst complex was fading from local memory, the campus itself was soon to be discovered in a new and deeply complicating way. Some years after Pennhurst's closure, an emerging recreational trend called "urban exploration" (UE) gained growing popularity among young people, thrill seekers, and curious adventure seekers of all types.

Urban exploration is the act of seeking out and physically exploring man-made places that are not often seen, or are off-limits to the public.

Abandoned places are very popular venues for this line of recreational activity: industrial sites; storm, sewer, and railroad tunnels; military installations; and abandoned institutions are all enticing targets. The act of UE is defended by proponents and practitioners as a form of urban archaeology, a lay person's means of exploring the past.

The presence of UE at closed institutions is quite commonplace. These are typically old, ornate, intrinsically foreboding structures—made all the more so by decades of films utilizing them as scenes of horror. They are natural sites for youthful exploration designed to test courage and seek thrills. Pennhurst, however, stands out because it acquired the reputation of being one of the "hottest" spots for paranormal activity in the country.

According to Jeff Chapman, the hobby of urban exploration is described as "a sort of interior tourism that allows the curious-minded to discover . . . places not designed for public usage. . . . [U]rban explorers strive to actually create authentic experiences [by] . . . appreciat[ing] fantastic, obscure places that might otherwise go completely neglected." Exploring abandoned buildings is a major focus of UE hobbyists, as Chapman directly addresses in a further definition. "Speaking broadly, urban exploration consists of seeking out, visiting and documenting interesting human-made spaces, most typically abandoned buildings."[2]

Chapman is credited in many UE circles as one of the key founders of the hobby. This Toronto-based adventurer established the website infiltration.org, in which he chronicled his own adventures, posted advice on "infiltration" (his name for urban exploration), and hosted online forums for other enthusiasts of the hobby. The book, completed shortly before he died of cancer at age thirty-two, was a compendium of the best knowledge on the website. With chapter topics like "Sneaking," "Abandoned Sites," and subchapter topics of "Moving Stealthily," "Alarms," and "Fast Talking," the book candidly and playfully explores the hobby extensively. *Access All Areas* is embraced by many in the UE community as a definitive handbook for the practice.

The hobby of UE is an informal pursuit, not an activity sanctioned or regulated by any authority or consortium. The recreation is practiced by individuals or small groups acting independently, similar to other groups of enthusiasts, like skateboarders or flash mobs. Given that UE involves the pursuit of "human-made spaces," specifically abandoned buildings, trespassing is often a vital component of the practice. Like many who engaged in the hobby, Chapman used an alias (*Ninjalicious*) for this very reason, to mitigate the legal risks involved with chronic trespassing.

Given that trespassing is often the only way to access a location of interest, the hobby exists on the fringes of legality. For this reason, Chapman stressed the importance of strictly followed a code of ethics for urban explorers. Certainly an outsider to the hobby can't help but be struck by the irony that ethics would weigh significantly into a hobby that relies on the systematic legal violation of trespassing. However Chapman's view follows a unique philosophical logic. "Beyond the 'do not enter' signs and out of the protected zone," he wrote, "you and your friends are free to behave as you really are . . . a lot of people who usually behave well do so because they're mindlessly obeying rules and laws. . . . People who think laws are more important than ethics are exactly the sorts who will wander into an abandoned area and be so confused by their sudden freedom and lack of supervision they'll start breaking windows and urinating on the floor."[3]

It is from this perspective that Chapman insists that a proper interpretation of the practice of UE is one that depends on a strict adherence to an ethical approach to the locations visited. "The broader urban exploration community has quite wisely adopted the Sierra Club's motto of 'take nothing but pictures, leave nothing but footprints.'" Chapman goes on later to implore that even footprints are too much to leave, especially when "infiltrating" an environment with active security.[4]

While the practice of UE regularly involves trespassing, in a pure interpretation of the hobby, the motives of such actors are often driven primarily by curiosity and genuine interest in understanding the purpose and history of a site through firsthand observation. Individuals with an interest in photography are common among UE groups. Photographing sites of exploration is a large part of the UE experience, often with the intention of sharing those images through websites dedicated to the pursuit of UE activities.

Chapman asserted on his website, "I don't think there is anything wrong with urban exploration, at least not the type described here. . . . Genuine urban explorers never vandalize, steal or damage anything—we don't even litter. We're in it for the thrill of discovery and a few nice pictures." Despite Chapman's claims, there is an undeniable dualism in the practice of UE. The self-enforced respect for a visited environment is offset by the means used to access that environment. Under the heading of "Ethics" on Chapman's website, he specifically addresses the topic of trespassing in somewhat glib terms. "Often all that lies between a merry band of infiltrators [explorers] and exploration paradise is a simple, two-dimensional warning sign. A warning sign that cruelly informs all who gaze upon it that . . . what lies behind the sign is too good for them. . . . [O]ur explorers have never signed any document agreeing to obey all signs they may encounter."[5]

Certainly the attitude expressed on the topic by Chapman is characterized by a sense of fun, but his logic betrays a disquieting philosophical contradiction. He proposes that rules are to be disregarded provided that an individual or group properly regulates itself, that the ends of visiting a neglected location justify the means required to access the location. However, the reality is that just as Chapman's followers signed no statement promising they would "obey all signs," so too they signed no agreement obligating them to follow his ascribed ethics, either.

Given that UE began in a fog of illegality, the activity will likely have a draw for followers who are comfortable, if not finding it preferable, operating outside of the law. In providing individuals the knowledge and encouragement to "infiltrate" an abandoned environment, ethically lax followers can just as easily disregard Chapman's moral consideration along with the "No Trespassing" sign they ignore. This is a dangerous combination for an abandoned location with no active policing.

Judging by the volume of video postings on YouTube and other internet sites, abandoned state institutions are a boon to UE enthusiasts, many of whom are young and disguise their identities by wearing hoodies and masks. The Pennhurst campus was discovered by UE enthusiasts at the turn of the twenty-first century. The expansion and scope of the internet as a forum for sharing accounts and photographs taken of the arresting state school complex only worked to accelerate the awareness and allure of Pennhurst State School as a place to explore. Internet UE forums rapidly filled with images and firsthand accounts of the buildings and their eerily forgotten contents.

"Abandoned Steve" and "Panda Princess" are two of the most popular UE sites on YouTube.[6] Images of decaying structures and interior rooms in disarray heightened the sense of eerie and forbidden grounds. Commentators remarked about supposed paranormal phenomenon, everything from seeing ghosts to hearing voices and "screams and moaning." On her visit in 1989, "Christine" claimed to hear voices coming from within one of the buildings, only to be assured by security guards people had left years before. Still photos and video of Embreeville State School revealed deplorable buildings and grounds, though the voice-over made clear the explorers had no understanding of where they were. "Insanely cool," declared the filmmaker.[7]

An urban explorer using the pseudonym "Marita" spoke to the allure of Pennhurst in the early days of its discovery by UE enthusiasts. Marita grew up close to the grounds of Philadelphia State Psychiatric Hospital at Byberry, commonly referred to as "Byberry." As a teenager she spent time exploring the empty campus and abandoned buildings of Byberry with her friends. Being an avid and skilled photographer, she took many pictures of the location in an effort to document the deteriorating campus.

It was in her senior year of high school that Marita first went to the Pennhurst Campus. She and her photography friends had heard of it through word of mouth, among other UE enthusiasts. It bears noting that while there are many UE websites where hobbyists share information about exploration sites, word of mouth is a vital mode of sharing site information and tips about locations.

Marita describes that first visit to Pennhurst as remarkable in how "pristine" the abandoned campus and buildings were. The location was eerie and haunting in those days because everything was undisturbed, left exactly as it had been when the doors had been locked years before. Excited by the discovery, and the many remarkable photographic opportunities found on the campus, Marita and her friends made repeated visits to the Pennhurst campus.

Moving from building to building, they captured images of an institutional life suspended in time; rooms and equipment set up for daily use, toys lying where they had last seen play, patient records sitting atop desks in nurses stations. In those early years of Pennhurst exploration by UE enthusiasts, the campus was literally a time capsule, sealed in 1987 and available for the discovery as a reward for breaking a lock or finding an unlatched window.

Word of Pennhurst's eerie wonders spread far and wide. Marita remembers encountering UE enthusiasts from all over the eastern United States exploring the site. One explorer she remembers specifically was a videographer who had traveled all the way from Florida specifically to shoot video of the abandoned state school.

The internet notoriety of Pennhurst through UE sites carried an effect that was also decidedly dualistic in nature and consequence. Through the UE websites the vast grounds and buildings of Pennhurst were effectively "rediscovered" by a public that knew little of the history or past of the campus. Some of the images of Pennhurst made by photographers exploring the site are arrestingly beautiful and emotive.

Unlike other sites devoted to Pennhurst, author Chris Peecho's Pennhurst page is dedicated to engendering healing and remembrance of the history of Pennhurst, and it is responsible for creating broader public awareness of the nature of institutionalization in the twentieth century.[8] Rich in detail and documentary resources, Peecho's work became one of the principal factors in the growing urge to preserve and protect the memory of what happened to people at Pennhurst. In this sense, it was a powerful positive force for awareness and historic understanding.

By comparison, most other internet websites featuring Pennhurst are ignorant of the campus's important role in the history of disability civil rights, promoting instead sensationalism and distortion that appeal to urban explorers seeking daredevil thrills. These websites instead recast the complex into the stuff of lurid urban legend. It is through these sites that a projected, fictionalized narrative began to emerge that swiftly subverted the meaning of Pennhurst and its importance to history in the eyes of an unknowing public.

## From the Historical to the Haunted

As Pennhurst's reputation grew as a prime location for urban exploration, so too did an alternate history begin to emerge. Amateur snapshots and posted web videos of the complex's moldering buildings, halls, and rooms rapidly appeared online under headings of "Abandoned Haunted Insane Asylum" and similar titles. A youthful audience of thrill seekers began to pour onto the campus to explore the "abandoned mental hospital." Without ready access to accurate information about the complex, or its important role in history, the campus was a blank slate free for projection. Without so much as a plaque to offer even a modest explanation of the site, these unofficial visitors were left to interpret Pennhurst with their imaginations, based solely on what they observed.

Marita speaks to this ambiguity of the apparent purpose of the Pennhurst complex. Wandering in the empty wards, explorers viewed toys, cribs, and child-sized wheelchairs. Most notable were the colorful hand-painted murals on the walls in many of the rooms depicting clowns, animals, and other juvenile themes. Marita and other explorers viewed these finds and assumed the facility was a children's hospital of some form. It was not—Pennhurst at the end had very few children.

The gothic atmosphere of the deteriorating and unlit setting led many to make very sinister interpretations of the facility. This was captured in many pictures posted to the UE websites. One particularly vivid example is an image of a child's wheelchair, lost in a dark basement room, set against a hand-painted candy-striped pillar. The photographer titled this poignant and haunting image "Candy Stripe Prison."

In the scope of such surroundings, it is easy to understand how an alternate narrative could quickly surface and take root. Given the rundown condition of the property, a gothic interpretation of Pennhurst is understandable, however inaccurate. Moreover, these conditions of the Pennhurst complex could lead a visitor to assume the location to be haunted, if the visitor were so inclined.

This belief of a haunted campus was driven in no small part by ample physical evidence of forced confinement of the former residents on the site: restraint straps, straitjackets, and windows covered with heavy steel security screens. These elements presented a narrative of implied horror and suffering that was self-evident, requiring no further interpretation or reference to actual history. Furthermore, the suffering that had occurred within the walls of Pennhurst was absolutely real; lives had been arrested at the school and in some cases lost, due to abuse and neglect. Drawing from this pervasively dark atmosphere on the abandoned campus, reports of paranormal activity at Pennhurst flourished, with the resulting attendant activities and attention. Unofficial ghost hunting and séances, among other activities of occult pursuit, became common occurrences on the abandoned grounds.

## Visitors of Another Kind

Chapman's approach, as expressed through his writings, tended toward a fun-loving, anarchic spirit. "There's something of a moral duty to explore abandoned sites. If you don't go and appreciate those beautiful places of decay, it's possible that no one will and that would be a terrible shame."[9] However, this freewheeling attitude is contrasted against a firmly advocated sense of ethics and responsibility. His concern for sites being forgotten by neglect is equally focused on concern in the opposite direction.

Chapman expressed a keen awareness of the responsibility that knowledge of such sites carried. Sharing information of interesting sites is an important part of UE culture, as evidenced by the prevalence of UE internet sites and related forums. However, breaking from his usual irreverent tone, he warns in his book of the importance of good judgment and discretion with sharing that information. "Giving the general public too much of the wrong sort of information (say, on a public website or a zine [niche magazine]) can make a site more attractive and vulnerable to people who aren't primarily motivated by the urge to explore, such as vandals looking for tunnels to tag in, partiers looking for a building where they can hold a rave, or thieves looking for a building to plunder."

Nowhere was this more true than on the Pennhurst campus. Not only were the curious drawn to the state school, but vandals were increasingly attracted to the campus as the years advanced. The walls of the buildings inside and out became message boards of competing graffiti. Windows and doors were systematically broken, and equipment left behind in the buildings was stolen or destroyed. At one point in the early part of this century, vandals set a fire in an upstairs office of the Administration Building. The building was damaged but not destroyed, as the local fire department responded in time.

Marita describes two very separate groups who frequented the campus in those times. There were the explorers, like her, who were drawn to the state school because it was a unique historic environment. The other "group" was the "partiers," as she described them, who also frequented the grounds and buildings. These "partiers" valued the campus for its freedoms, wherein they could do as they pleased, be that to consume alcohol, engage in recreational drug use, or commit widespread acts of vandalism. Marita draws a direct connection between a destructive surge in the visitation of the partiers and the completed demolition of Byberry Psychiatric Hospital at around the same time. The same tags and telltale vandalism that had blighted Byberry began appearing in abundance at Pennhurst. In the absence of Byberry, these partiers and vandals presumably now frequented Pennhurst, bringing their spray paint, matches, and hammers with them.

An atmosphere of anarchy and physical violence began to pervade the empty complex. The state-issued "No Trespassing" signs were of little function, as no authority from the Commonwealth of Pennsylvania enforced the order. This condition of lawlessness coincided with a surge in the world economy, especially the demand for raw materials in rapidly growing, emerging economies like China and India. The market for scrap metal became remarkably profitable, and with this incentive, the old campus became a target for scrap metal thieves.

In the space of a few years, in the mid-2000s, scrappers, as the thieves are sometimes called, stripped the central kitchen of its kettles and fittings and literally yanked copper wiring and plumbing from the walls of buildings. In a shocking act of blatant thievery, scrappers tore the copper skin from the iconic grand cupola atop the Administration

Building. This verdigris structure, topped by an elegant wind vane, was an architectural feature of the campus visible from almost every building on the complex. The campus was known for this decorative feature.

The theft of the cupola skin is a remarkable and ironic example of the dualistic role played by the internet during this stage of Pennhurst's history. Individuals who stole the copper skin were as uncouth as they were brazen and shot a video of their kleptomaniacal exploits. The stolen copper skins were recovered by the police, but without any public authority representing Pennhurst, the police had no one to whom to return the stolen property. Ultimately, the panels were sold for scrap, melted down and lost forever. In the end the cupola was left standing and stripped, rusting iron beams supporting a disembodied copper roof.

This destructive and anarchic period may have hit its deepest inflection point sometime in 2008 or 2009. Marita relays a story about another significant act of violation against the historic campus. In that era on the Pennhurst campus, among the UE set and the partiers alike, there was an unofficial agreement concerning a set of terracotta murals on the Administrative Building.

These ceramic murals, images of workers laboring in fields, were crafted in the Great Depression as part of a Works Progress Administration art project for the beautification of the state school. The collective agreement among those who frequented the abandoned campus was that these murals were strictly off limits for any sort of theft, vandalism, or defacement. Windows could be broken, copper could be stolen, walls could be tagged with spray paint and artifacts could be stolen, but the murals were to remain untouched.

This unofficial pact was violated when vandals attacked the three-dimensional murals with hammers and defaced the figures depicted in the images with spray paint. Marita describes the collective outcry of the many unofficial groups, with their divergent motivations, who frequented Pennhurst in those times. The online forums lit up with expressions of collective outrage over this violation of the campus. Threats were openly made against the perpetrators, should they be discovered, and there was a collective realization among these many camps that Pennhurst was vulnerable and needed to be protected. Some individuals even heeded this late call by scrubbing away graffiti on the campus they had sprayed themselves.

Marita describes the damage to these murals as a significant turning point. The collective sense of violation created by the act generated unification among many groups and individuals not previously inclined to collective thinking. In some ways the sad incident established a sense of society among many who could be described as antisocial. This collective realization of the vulnerability of Pennhurst and its need for protection came far too late. The damage to the buildings at the hands of vandals and scrappers was extensive. What had once been untouched and eerily pristine, those elements treasured by the UE community, was now thoroughly looted and ravaged with destruction. The urban exploration era had effectively ended at Pennhurst.

The discovery and opening of the Pennhurst complex to the public by the UE community was decidedly dualist in its outcome. Through online postings and word of mouth, the campus became well known to the UE community. In fact, this was true of numerous abandoned institutional sites that had fallen into disrepair. The attention worked to raise awareness of the campus and, in constructive hands, taught the site's true history and importance. In the long run the attention of UE enthusiasts influenced disability rights advocates while encouraging more purposeful preservation of the buildings and grounds. By contrast that same public awareness brought by UE interests drew thrill seekers, vandals, and thieves.

Like the copper cupola, the emblematic crown of the campus, Pennhurst was heisted both physically and symbolically while no one was watching. Ultimately, the significance of this cradle of the civil rights movement for citizens with intellectual and developmental disabilities has been tainted by exploitation and now commercial development. The symbol of the place has been hijacked and used for quick profit, at both the detriment of the physical place, but more significantly, to the meaning of the cause that made the site historically significant.

As with the UE trend, however, the sword has two edges. The influx of money from the Pennhurst Asylum has permitted the owner to stabilize some of the buildings that would otherwise certainly have decayed to the point beyond repair. That is a very positive outcome from the point of view of architectural preservation. What remains is the preservation of the dignity of the lives of the more than 10,600 people who lived on these grounds.

The future of the Pennhurst State School and Hospital complex hangs precariously in the shifting balance between the capitalistic exploits of its current owner and the desire for preservation and historical accuracy among advocates and preservationists. How this uncertainty will find conclusion is unknown. The advocates work exhaustedly with limited resources to correct this devastation of the campus and its symbolic meaning, while successive private owners seek new ways to make a profitable return on their investment in real estate. The latest commercial scheme includes demolition to make way for an industrial park and is aided by a multimillion-dollar government aid package.

Without significant assistance to the cause of the advocates, either by private endowments or government assistance, the future of the campus and its known legacy hold little promise. Just as the rain continues to drip through the remaining structures of Pennhurst, so too does the willful exploitation of public ignorance of Pennhurst's meaning bring ruin both to the structure and the legacy of Pennhurst State School and Hospital.

## Notes

1. This "New Pennhurst" was a program from the 1960s to remake the institution and bring it up to modern standards.

2. Jeff Chapman, *Access All Areas: A User's Guide to the Art of Urban Exploration* (Toronto: Infilpress, 2005), 3; see also chapter 3. Chapman went by pen name "Ninjalicious."

3. Ibid., 19.

4. Ibid., 20.

5. "Warning Signs: A Guide to Ignoring Them by Ninjalicious," Infiltration, http://www.infiltration.org/ethics-warning.html.

6. "Abandoned Pennhurst State School and Hospital," YouTube, https://www.youtube.com/watch?v=mHgBodHnAUM.

7. "Embreeville Complex," Abandoned Exploration, https://abandonedexplorersite.wordpress.com/2017/05/01/embreevillecomplex; "Abandoned Embreeville State Hospital Complex Walkthrough," YouTube, https://www.youtube.com/watch?v=5Non8d9q_w4.

8. http://www.elpeecho.com/pennhurst/pennhurst.htm.

9. Chapman, *Access All Areas*, 89.

CHAPTER 10

# Preservation

*A Case Study of Collective Conscience*

NATHANIEL GUEST

The struggle to preserve Pennhurst was in a way reinvigorated by the era of urban exploration and its pernicious manifestations of partying, gang-like competition, and destruction. Outrage against that nihilistic use of the grounds helped give rise to a new emergence of concern for respectful memory and preservation. It would eventually take the form of a new nonprofit, the Pennhurst Memorial and Preservation Alliance, mandated not just to save a collection of buildings but to create a repository of memory.

But accelerating decay, insensitive, incompatible uses, vandalism, and bureaucratic neglect threatened the buildings. As a physical asset and as a moral and emotional space, Pennhurst faced a future that on all counts was uncertain at best. Failure to adequately consider Pennhurst both as a physical resource and as a watershed moment in the evolution of our culture may be as deep and far-reaching as the willful blindness of the institution's past.

In 1969, there were 290 public institutions like Pennhurst in the United States; today there are only about 140.[1] Pennhurst in this sense is just one of about 170 public institutions for people with intellectual and developmental disabilities that have closed over the past forty-five years.

Pennhurst does, of course, stand out because of its remarkably pivotal role in establishing positive social changes in the disability rights movement—the right to education, the right to treatment, the right to live in the community—but its fate does raise the question: how is America to remember the deplorable eugenics and institutional phase of our history, if the physical locations are all destroyed or repurposed? Are museums enough, without the raw emotional impact of the huge isolated *places* themselves?

Despite their decaying and overgrown appearance, Pennhurst's buildings were built for the millennia. With even a modicum of maintenance, the buildings could have lasted centuries. Simple expediency would have counseled that any plans for Pennhurst would need to address reuse of nearly six hundred thousand square feet of exceedingly well-built building stock as a first priority. If logic did not so counsel, one would have hoped that the law would.

In 1986, the Pennsylvania Historical and Museum Commission (PHMC) declared the property eligible for the National Register of Historic Places. Under the Pennsylvania History Code, the Commonwealth was under a legal mandate to provide for the property's maintenance and appropriate disposition. By the time Pennhurst officially closed in 1987, the Commonwealth had had nearly a decade to make such plans. As of 1988, when Pennhurst's campus was declared surplus property by the Department of Public Welfare and transferred to the Department of General Services (DGS), no plan for the buildings and their maintenance, reuse, or preservation had been forthcoming.

Years of neglect, confusion, and bureaucratic inaction clouded the preservation process at Pennhurst. To this day, nomination to the National Register has not occurred. For twenty years after its closing, no one made the effort. Since its sale, nomination is not in the private owner's interest due to imposition of potent restrictions on property use and reuse. Pennhurst closed in 1987, and there was a clear pattern of state and local confusion from 1988 to 2008. During those years, the fate of Pennhurst's historic core of approximately seventeen buildings, 125 acres of once-manicured landscape, and 1,600 feet of Schuylkill River frontage fell to well-intentioned, if ultimately misguided, local entities that tried to fill the void in the absence of state leadership. In 2008, the property's sale to a private investment group, Pennhurst Acquisitions, was finally consummated.

The story of the Pennhurst institution offers an extremely informative "case study" of the degree to which state laws and regulations regarding preservation of historically important properties can be ignored. The Commonwealth had a duty within its own legal structure to maintain the buildings and grounds to maintain its value—for use, reuse, or preservation. This duty was ignored across several gubernatorial administrations.

While the owners say they are open to preservation, they cite the condition of the buildings as a limiting factor. The degradation of Pennhurst's buildings in the period of state ownership after closure and prior to their sale violated Pennsylvania's History Code. Moreover, DGS's transfer of the site out of public ownership without notifying PHMC was a History Code violation equivalent to a slap in the face to the preservation community.[2] According to the PHMC Bureau of Historic Preservation staff and the National Trust for Historic Preservation, violations of the History Code seen at Pennhurst are emblematic of major problems in the disposition of state historic property. Even when the PHMC recommends preservation easements on historic properties, other state agencies do not follow that recommendation—just as DGS failed to do with Pennhurst. In the absence of state-level protection or federal involvement, properties are left to the mercy of local-level protections.

Local politics can be a dominant factor in these stories. One of the most remarkable political facets of the Pennhurst property history took place in 2007 and 2008, when East Vincent Board of Supervisors Chairman Ryan Costello first approved proposals and waivers for reuse without revelation of any specific plans, then resigned from the board. He became the Pennhurst Acquisitions attorney, and then advocated for *very* favorable and flexible rezoning before that same board—and succeeded in 2012. In 2014, Mr. Costello ran for the U.S. House of Representatives seat vacated by Jim Gerlach, and won the seat.

Pennhurst has a modicum of protection under East Vincent Township's preservation ordinances. However, the Township has indicated it has no intention of interpreting the ordinance to require preservation of a significant portion of the site—if indeed any—if it is against the property owner's wishes.[3] Moreover, a letter from the National Trust for Historic Preservation in May 2009 reminding the Township of the fact that their demolition by neglect provisions were being repeatedly violated by Pennhurst's owner was met with hostility.

Absent a preservation easement or unusually proactive local involvement, there was no mechanism to ensure the property's survival posttransfer—a point made painfully clear at Pennhurst when, just months after the transfer, the campus's priceless Depression-era tile mosaics were vandalized. According to the National Trust for Historic Preservation, Pennsylvania is not alone. Deficient protections for historic state properties plus the challenges of reusing large institutions mean that precious few places like Pennhurst have been saved.

## Creating the Pennhurst Memorial and Preservation Alliance (PMPA)

The idea of preservation began with a tour of the Pennhurst campus Greg Pirmann[4] and I had taken in 2007. The Alliance grew in 2008 when Greg and I reached out to Chris Cadwalader, webmaster for a Pennhurst-oriented website. Together, we three fashioned a presentation for the local historical society, an event that sparked an overwhelming response. Nearly three hundred people packed the assembly hall. Pennhurst meant a great deal to many people in the area, yet they could not really talk about it until this event made it possible. As a result, the Pennhurst Memorial and Preservation Alliance was formed.

Later that year, the website www.preservepennhurst.org was launched, based on Cadwalader's extensive scholarly work. With frequent updates, large photographic and video archives, and blogs to share stories and comments, it has become the definitive website about Pennhurst. Indeed, the site also hosted information about the deinstitutionalization effort that followed the struggle over Pennhurst. An interactive timeline added in 2010 has been cited in several academic works.

The founding members of the PMPA responded to more requests for presentations in the Spring City / Royersford / Pottstown area from churches, historical societies, and business leagues. As word spread, the coalition grew from just a few local activists to nearly forty leaders in the disability rights, historic preservation, and development world. Joining the group were Ginny Thornburgh, former first lady of Pennsylvania and disability advocate, as well as Thomas Gilhool, Esq., the attorney who took the *Pennhurst* case to the United States Supreme Court three times, and former NBC 10 reporter Bill Baldini, whose 1968 documentary *Suffer the Little Children* thrust Pennhurst into the national spotlight.

Dr. James Conroy joined the group upon its incorporation in 2009 and serves as its copresident along with Jean M. Searle, a Pennhurst class member. Conroy was the investigator and designer of the Pennhurst Longitudinal Study that is described in chapter 8. Ms. Searle grew up in institutions in and near Scranton, far from her Philadelphia family, and was scheduled to be moved to Pennhurst at age twenty-two. However, because of Judge Broderick's 1978 Order, admissions to Pennhurst were closed. Instead, she moved to a small group home in Philadelphia. She has since moved to her own apartment and has held a good job with the Disability Rights Network advocacy agency for twenty-four years. She is a member of many of the state's most influential boards of directors in the disability field and is a speaker at local, state, and national venues.

Since 2008, PMPA staff have offered dozens of programs on the history of the disability rights movement and the need to preserve Pennhurst as a repository of memory and a locus of action for the future. PMPA programs have been structured to inform, to gather information, and to encourage participants to share their stories. Each program asks participants to think critically about Pennhurst's history, asking questions like: "What happened there?" "How did society allow such neglect to happen in our own backyard?" "How did a grassroots effort galvanize such sweeping social change?" and "What should happen at the Pennhurst campus to respectfully remember and positively add to our region?"

Through PMPA efforts, Pennhurst has been recertified for eligibility to the National Register of Historic Places. It has been on the Most Endangered lists for both Preservation Pennsylvania and the Preservation Alliance of Greater Philadelphia. It was included in the National Trust for Historic Preservation's This Place Matters campaign. The PMPA's early advocacy efforts have been highlighted by several websites and print publications, including the *Philadelphia Inquirer*, the *Pottstown Mercury*, and the *West Chester Daily Local*.

In 2010, an official historical marker from the Pennsylvania Historical and Museum Commission was dedicated to Pennhurst and placed on a highway outside the Pennhurst campus. The PMPA worked with the Public Interest Law Center of Philadelphia to plan and fund a day-long conference and dedication ceremony entitled *Triumph and Tragedy: Telling the Pennhurst Story*. In partnership with the Law Center, the PMPA obtained a $3,000 grant from the Pennsylvania Humanities Council, Pennsylvania's affiliate with the National Endowment for the Humanities. A large fundraising effort paid for the event in full, allowing the day's activities to be offered to the public free of charge.

A conference in conjunction with the marker dedication brought the current leaders and early pioneers in the disability advocacy field back to Pennhurst—where their movement scored its first and most momentous victory—for the first time in many decades. The event was an opportunity for the general public to see, hear, and meet those associated with Pennhurst—the residents, the employees, the families, and those working to secure a better future outside of institutional walls. Similarly, it was a chance for various Pennhurst communities to meet each other again, or perhaps for the first time. Given the age of those with firsthand Pennhurst experience, the PMPA understood that the dedication ceremony would likely be the last time an event such as this would be possible. They used the event to begin video recording stories for a future archive of life stories—which will become part of interactive exhibits about the disability rights movement and Pennhurst.

The cathartic value of this event cannot be underestimated. As thousands of emails to PMPA attest, there is a great need within our various communities, particularly among those who lived and worked at Pennhurst and their families, to share their experiences, things they have not felt comfortable talking about in other venues. The commemoration brought those people together and honored their struggle.

## The Case for Preservation

Where the meaning of a historic place is contested, the mandate to preserve it for future consideration becomes all the more important. A cultural landscape reflects a society's feelings, as well as its needs, thoughts, values, and memories. Whether under construction, in use, reuse, disuse, or abandonment, a cultural landscape is the visual record of processes and relationships at work within a society. Cultural landscapes created for a given set of needs can become irrelevant when those needs change. But, even in disuse, they can become icons, representing events and ideology that over time are either revered or despised. So it is with Pennhurst.

Even within the disability community, Pennhurst is both reviled and treasured. It can be remembered as the site of unspeakable pain and horror so that we may never go back there again. It also can serves as a memorial to great triumphs in the disability rights movement.

Amidst the poles of meaning, one thing is undeniable: a tour of the property itself yields tremendous emotional impact. This is a town-sized "colony," built specifically to isolate and segregate a portion of our own citizens. One cannot visit the place itself without evoking wonder—how did that happen, why did it happen, can we prevent it from happening ever again? And therein lies a great value of preservation.

Pennhurst has been designated an International Site of Conscience,[5] one of over two hundred locations in a "global network of historic sites, museums and memory initiatives" connecting past and present struggles for "human rights and social justice." Dedicated to historical memory and preservation, each of these sites is recognized as a worthy candidate for a master plan of preservation and reuse. Like the master plan for the preservation of the Auschwitz concentration camp site,[6] advocates see Pennhurst as a critically important place in twentieth-century history. It must be a place of remembrance that can be visited, experienced, and integrated into a collective historical and moral conscience.

## Preserving Buildings as Memory

Pennhurst's built landscape must be used to tell the story on the actual Pennhurst grounds. Pennhurst should be a place of memory and reflection guided by the buildings themselves.

The connection of buildings with memory is as old as written history. The use of a building as a memory reference can be traced to Simonides of Greece in the fifth and sixth century BC, who envisioned storytelling from memory as a walk through a temple. Each element of the temple form, from foundation to roof, became a reminder where memorized spatial relationships established memories translated into story. Japanese tradition uses a "memory palace" in much the same way. The memory palace technique became prized in Japan by students of law struggling to remember a vast array of unwritten canons.[7]

While such "memory palaces" house a particular set of thoughts, most buildings, including those at Pennhurst, are designed for more common purposes. Seeing how the buildings were laid out, with large dormitory sleeping quarters, huge "dayrooms," and no food facilities (meals were brought in on trays from a "Dietary" building), brings home with great power the extent to which these institutions were *not* designed to be "homes" or "home-like." Instead, they were places of warehousing and efficiency, based on treating people *en masse*, along the command and control models of the day. Individual identities were submerged in the architecture itself.

Now that the historic core of Pennhurst is privately owned, the question becomes: How can the buildings be reused in an economically sustainable way and still tell the essential Pennhurst story?

In 2010, the Pennhurst Memorial and Preservation Alliance partnered with the Preservation Alliance for Greater Philadelphia to apply for a reuse design and feasibility study grant. The study, sponsored by the Community Design Collaborative (CDC),[8] included, among other things, a design charrette and community meetings. These meetings provided ideas for and noted concerns that enhanced a series of three market studies then underway by the Cornell University Program in Real Estate. Preliminary recommendations from the Cornell studies, in turn, guided the CDC design team. The Urban Partners firm of Philadelphia unofficially participated in the study and provided early guidance on economic feasibility.

The CDC's work helped to refine the idea of a "community of conscience" at Pennhurst in keeping with its designation as an International Site of Conscience. They gathered public and professional input on what uses such a community might include and channeled that input into two reuse design scenarios.

The first contemplated a self-sufficient, green lifestyle community with some degree of self-sufficiency. Green communities across the nation appear in a variety of shades, usually differentiated by the type and scope of programming around environmental issues. The team felt that Pennhurst offered opportunities to showcase recommended practices in building technologies, adaptive reuse, agriculture, energy conservation and passive production, storm water management, and possibly transportation/circulation. All restoration and new construction, they offered, should focus on sustainability.

The second scenario capitalized on what the design team saw as strong potential for educational reuse. Based in part on public input from the PMPA's website, the design team postulated that prime educational opportunities could include arts and trades training, a business incubation and employment center, demonstration agriculture, and a green technologies incubator. The site might also become a conference center, a college, or trade school. This scenario included possible reuse as a museum or venue for art and culture.

However, both scenarios essentially erased any negative history associated with the site. That is exactly what happened to Pineland Farms in Maine. Moreover, at the time of the work, the 2008 economic recession in the United States made major development projects of this kind very unlikely—and very hard to finance.

To the dismay of the disability advocacy community, the financially lucrative Pennhurst Asylum Halloween amusement park still exploits imagery and storylines that are extremely hurtful and degrading to the memory of people with disabilities. Chapter 11 makes this abundantly clear. Another impediment appeared in 2018 when Derek Strine, who had purchased the property, secured a $4 million grant and other loan securities from the Commonwealth to further his plans to erect a large commercial and industrial park on the former campus. Buildings have been demolished to make way for the enterprise, and although the Asylum venue was not affected, the new development poses risks to any museum or suitable memorial.[9]

As much as advocates would like to partner with the owners of the property to construct memorials, monuments, plaques, a walking trail, guided tours, and historically accurate history museum displays, this is simply not possible while the property is being used in a way that makes people with disabilities into monsters and objects of terror.

The PMPA's position is that over the next few years the owners will realize that *just as much money can be made from a Halloween attraction that does not use disability imagery*. The nearby Eastern State Penitentiary in Philadelphia conducts both Halloween events and year-round historic tours, and the enterprise does not employ horrific depictions of guards and prisoners to make it one of the most popular venues on the east coast. When the Pennhurst owners eventually arrive at a similar respectful point, a strong and enduring partnership will be feasible. Pennhurst can become a symbol of our disability history, and can serve as a model and stepping stone for what the PMPA Board believes is inevitable: a national memorial and museum in Washington commemorating the disability rights movement in America.

## Notes

1. S. A. Larson, P. Salmi, D. Smith, L. Anderson, and A. S. Hewitt, *Residential Services for Persons with Intellectual or Developmental Disabilities: Status and Trends Through 2011* (Minneapolis: University of Minnesota, Research and Training Center on Community Living, Institute on Community Integration, 2013).

2. PMPA, " Pennhurst Timeline" Pennhurst Memorial and Preservation Alliance, http://www.preservepennhurst.org/default.aspx?pg=93.

3. The final agreement of sale of Pennhurst to Mr. Richard Chakejian's group was obtained by the author through a Freedom of Information Act request and included a

development proposal that would effectively eliminate the historic district entirely and place 240 single-family homes on the site.

4. J. Gregory Pirmann, author of chapter 2 and PMPA Vice President..

5. "Pennhurst Memorial and Preservation Alliance (USA)," International Coalition of Sites of Conscience, https://www.sitesofconscience.org/en/membership/pennhurst-memorial-and-preservation-alliance.

6. "Master Plan for Preservation," Auschwitz-Birkinau Memorial and Museum, http://auschwitz.org/en/museum/preservation/master-plan-for-preservation.

7. Jonathon Spence, *Memory Palace of Matteo Ricci* (New York: Penguin Books, 1985).

8. The CDC is a volunteer-based center that provides pro bono preliminary design services for nonprofit organizations in the Philadelphia region.

9. Jacob Adleman, "Notorious Pennhurst Hospital Campus Gets Pa. Grant Toward Rebirth as Business Park," *Philadelphia Inquirer*, November 21, 2017, https://www.inquirer.com/philly/business/real_estate/commercial/notorious-pennhurst-hospital-campus-gets-pa-grant-toward-rebirth-as-business-park-20171121.html.

CHAPTER 11

# The Final Indignity and the Dawning of Hope

EMILY SMITH BEITIKS

Ghosts are commonly believed to be the spirits of those who have unfinished business remaining in our mortal world. Many ghost stories tell of people with a tortured past who haunt the living so that they can pay back to others the harm done to them. Following this logic, high schoolers looking for a spooky Friday night and professional paranormal experts alike have headed to the site of the Pennhurst State School and Hospital since it was abandoned, for where could you find a more likely place to encounter such tortured souls?

During its years of operation, a total of over 10,600 people lived at Pennhurst, many passing their entire lives within its bounding walls. But like many institutions housing people with disabilities, Pennhurst eventually became a place of abuse and neglect. Two Supreme Court cases on behalf of Pennhurst residents, as well as a 1968 television news exposé by journalist Bill Baldini called *Suffer the Little Children*, helped bring these issues to light. Investigations in the late 1960s found that over 3,500 residents were living in Pennhurst with only six hundred workers to assist them, and that many staff were mistreating and sometimes physically harming the residents. There were cases in which residents were raped, sometimes while others watched and did not attempt to stop it. Residents who acted out were cruelly punished—one man was beaten repeatedly with a toilet bowl brush, leaving welts all over his body. Others were neglected, some left naked in beds or caged in cribs all day long.

If you believe in ghosts, then it is easy to believe that Pennhurst would be a haunted site. However, I wish to avoid assessing the verity of the paranormal. Instead, I explore a different type of haunting at Pennhurst: not that of the supernatural, but rather that of the history of abuses under institutionalization, now being rewritten through Pennhurst's current existence as a for-profit haunted house attraction, known as the Pennhurst Asylum. For the record, Pennhurst never was a psychiatric hospital or asylum, although it must be noted that people with mental illnesses are equally undeserving of disrespectful depictions in Halloween attractions.

How did this attraction come to be? Nearly twenty years after the horrific stories of abuse were made public, Pennhurst was finally shut down, and the residents were relocated into group homes. The property sat abandoned for years, with much of the equipment—wheelchairs, hospital beds, and medical devices—left behind. In February 2008, a group well educated about Pennhurst's past formed the Pennhurst Memorial and Preservation Alliance (PMPA), a nonprofit dedicated to making Pennhurst into a national museum. But standing in the way of PMPA's vision was a businessman named Richard Chakejian, who organized a group of private investors who purchased Pennhurst from the state for a little over $2 million.[1] He struggled to turn it into a money-making venture at the height of the nation's great economic downturn, with little success, until his teenager suggested that he capitalize on Pennhurst's frightful allure and convert it into a haunted house.[2] At the turn of the century, people with disabilities were often regarded as a threat to the social order. It was this fear that motivated Pennhurst's original construction and this same fear, fused with ignorance, insensitivity, and commercialism, that led to Pennhurst's September 2010 rebirth as Chakejian's "Pennhurst Asylum." New owner Derek Strine has continued this legacy.

Pennhurst is not the first haunted house to be set at a deinstitutionalized asylum or state school. But given the significant role that Pennhurst played in the deinstitutionalization movement—from the public attention captured by the news exposé to the two Supreme Court rulings—this attraction is of particular importance. PMPA made a public plea to Chakejian and Randy Bates, a local haunted house creator hired to design the attraction, to show respect for the history of Pennhurst. PMPA suggested that if a haunted house were hosted on the site, then it should be themed with vampires, Frankenstein's monsters, and the like rather than mental patients and people with disabilities. Chakejian assured PMPA and reporters that the request would be heeded, but when the attraction opened its doors to the public, the asylum connections were unavoidable, melded with a fictional legend of an Austrian scientist named "Dr. Chakajian" (an alternative spelling of Chakejian), whose experiments on prisoners went awry.[3] The result is a bizarre hybrid of history and legend, and of criminality and commercialism that simultaneously evokes and erases Pennhurst's troubled past.

The legend of "Dr. Chakajian" and his deranged, lab-rat prisoners is ostensibly meant to distance the Asylum from Pennhurst's history. Bates told a reporter from the *Philadelphia Inquirer*, "We created a backstory specifically to counteract any type of correlation between the former residents and what we're doing here."[4] Nonetheless, the attraction largely plays off, and often directly references, Pennhurst's actual history. On the Pennhurst Asylum website, Bates writes, "Not only does this place have an incredible ambience, a built-in cult following, and a treasure trove of unique props, it has a history; a history of mental patients chained to the walls in dark tunnels, children left for years in cribs, sexual abuse by the staff and even murder. . . . I am blown away by this scene. I can picture the thousands of customers coming through our attraction knowing that everything in here is REAL. My arms have gooseflesh!"[5]

A visit to the attraction actively weaves backstory and history.[6] In the long admission line, attendees pass a large movie screen that plays two films on a continuous loop: a condensed version of the news report *Suffer the Little Children* and a short video telling the story of "Dr. Chakajian" and his prison experiments, with images of actual lobotomies and footage that closely resembles that of the news report. Which video is fiction and which is reportage can be hard to tell. While waiting in line, the person next to me asked in earnest, "Is that real?" Perversely, *Suffer the Little Children* seems less credible in this context, and the legend more plausible.

The splicing together of history and legend continues throughout the attraction. The first rooms of the haunted house were set up as a museum exhibit in the hope of minimizing criticism. These rooms have an upbeat feel—they are brightly lit, music from the turn of the century plays, and pictures of the happier times at Pennhurst line the walls. However, attendees are moved through them quickly (something that many have complained about on the event's Facebook page), and completely staged elements filter into them, making it hard to distinguish museum from haunted house. Connecting two rooms in the museum, for example, is a dark passageway with a screen showing an actor playing a mental patient screaming for help in a locked room. The museum also includes an advertisement for the attraction itself—this is now part of Pennhurst's story.

In the haunted house, some rooms are no different from what you would find at any other haunted house, filled with corpses and bloody limbs, but other rooms and actor personas are directly inspired by Pennhurst's history. One room is made to look like the Pennhurst dormitory, and although the bodies are not seen—they are hidden under blankets, leaving visitors to wonder who will jump out where—they are reminiscent of the many motionless bodies seen in *Suffer the Little Children*, where people's muscles had atrophied from being confined too long in cage-like beds. Another room just looks like a disgusting bathroom—no animatronic surprises or actors jumping out, only a nod to the deplorable conditions of Pennhurst's past. Perhaps the most disturbing and direct Pennhurst references are rooms that depict the technology left behind when Pennhurst closed, including an old electric shock therapy machine and a dentist's chair that was reportedly used when teeth were pulled from unruly people living at Pennhurst.[7] The Pennhurst Asylum website itself points out that these artifacts are real and explains their use.

The actors portray evil doctors, nurses/aides, and patients. Granted, the caretakers as well as the patients are made to look evil—a departure from the trope in horror films and campfire urban legends of the marauding mental patient attacking innocent civilians. But this portrayal flattens out the actual power relations at Pennhurst, which were historically tipped quite dramatically: caretakers abused people who lived there. More accurate is the attraction slogan, repeated throughout the attraction, "The good doctor is always looking for new test subjects."

Chakejian defended the attraction by suggesting that because the majority of attendees are young, they do not know the history. (He argued that the brouhaha of activist groups who condemn the attraction is "what really brings up the horrors of the past." At the same time, he added, "Our kids are smart enough to understand the difference between reality and make-believe."[8] But sheer smarts are of no use if the information one gets is fundamentally wrong, and it is this that makes the Pennhurst Asylum's blurring of legend and history so misguided. The atrocities of torture and rape start to sound like ghost story clichés meant to enhance the thrill of the attraction, along the lines of the fabricated backstory used to promote *The Blair Witch Project*.[9]

In addition to how it misleads visitors, Pennhurst Asylum also feels, to many who were once residents there, deeply disrespectful. By representing itself as haunted only fictitiously, the promoters blithely forget that there are likely people haunted by Pennhurst and the many other institutions where abuses occurred. Jean Searle, copresident of PMPA and former resident of another institution, explains, "I don't want to relive the hell that I went through. I want to try to forget."[10]

In publicity materials for Pennhurst Asylum, Randy Bates encouraged attendees to put themselves in "patients'"[11] shoes. He suggested, "As you walk into these rooms, you can feel the air get heavy, the sounds deaden and you can imagine how the patients felt being locked up in the pitch dark with no one hearing your screams."[12] One could argue that this aims to foster empathy. Yet it seems more likely that this is another form of harm done to those who once resided at Pennhurst. Can someone attending a haunted attraction where actors may jump out at any moment actually contemplate the lifetimes of personal hardships that many Pennhurst residents experienced in a meaningful way? And if so, is it even accurate for attraction attendees to imagine Pennhurst as Bates described it, reducing residents' experiences to pure terror without acknowledging how many people also persisted and found the strength to carry on, despite facing horrific abuses each day? Bates frequently repeated this invitation for attendees to build a connection with the residents, but given the placement of this invitation within PR materials inviting attendees to the attraction, it is most likely that he prioritizes enhancing the experience of fear that leads to fun.

Bates's provocation that attendees identify with the people who lived at Pennhurst points to a bigger question: Can the haunted attraction provide a means of educating people about this often forgotten or unknown history? In an essay, bioethicist Dayle DeLancey writes: "'Haunted' hospital stories have been mainstays of U.S. television programs, feature films, and websites since the late 1990s. Medical ethicists and medical historians might be tempted to dismiss these depictions as mere vagaries of popular culture, but that would be an unfortunate oversight because haunted hospital lore memorializes historical claims of patient abuse, neglect, and maltreatment." DeLancey demonstrates that such ghost stories have merit through the case study of Danvers State Hospital, an abandoned site with an overlapping history to Pennhurst. She cites the work of historian Judith Richardson, who argues that ghosts "are produced by the cultural and social life of the communities in which they appear. . . . [and] operate as a particular, and peculiar, kind of social memory, an alternate form of history-making in which things usually forgotten, discarded, or repressed become foregrounded . . . as items of fear, regret, explanation, or desire."[13] Does the Pennhurst attraction deserve credit for publicizing an otherwise neglected past, as DeLancey argues with Danvers?

Pennhurst Asylum's purposeful blurring of myth and history make it hard to believe that any valuable history lesson can come from it. In fact, DeLancey also acknowledges a murkiness to the lore surrounding Danvers State Hospital, where many of the stories describing the haunted intertwine with accounts of witchcraft, due to the hospital's close proximity to Salem, Massachusetts. Two additional points draw out the distinctions between haunted hospital lore and the haunted asylum attraction that challenge the possibility that the attraction helps keep this history lesson present.

First, when history transitions into ghost stories, the presence of the supernatural distracts from the reality of the injustices committed. Both Danvers State Hospital and Pennhurst are said to be places where "evil things happened."[14] Yet "evilness" is not typically something that can be explained. Culturally, we associate it with the supernatural or the satanic to suggest that evil is a force existing outside of human control; we can succumb to it or resist it, but we cannot eliminate or even explain its unceasing presence. The horrific abuses that occurred commonly in state institutions for people with physical and mental disabilities, on the other hand, have been thoroughly explained. They resulted from a society that shunned people with disabilities and had not yet considered inclusion; a lack of funds and institutional support, making more adequate forms of care impossible with even the very best employees; and a widespread cultural, and in particular medical, ignorance about what was the best "treatment" for people with disabilities. To celebrate the ghost story fails to acknowledge the distortion that results when we focus in on a supernatural evil rather than man-made corruption.

The second reason complicating the notion that ghost stories memorialize the history of abuses for sites like Pennhurst is that since the 1990s, haunting has become an industry. Unlike Danvers State Hospital—not yet the site of such an attraction—Pennhurst and other similar locations have been overrun by commercial mechanisms that concoct the haunting stories, overwriting "social memory." While those who know about the Pennhurst attraction are likely to encounter the frequently repeated claim that "the fear is real," this language is a marketing gimmick, and Pennhurst's rewriting of history is indeed quite profitable in many configurations.

With slight alterations in imagery, current owner Strine has continued to play on the macabre, to huge financial benefit. In 2018, online testimonials included, "My experience was truly great. I caught two ghosts in my camera." Another visitor stated, "The place is awesome! Went last season and the new tunnels were amazing." "Fun holiday adventure," declared a third. Those posting noted the long lines and wait times of twenty to forty minutes, or more. The VIP and Combo Passes allowed you to skip the lines for a mere $78. Private ghost tours could range well over $1,000 according to the website.[15]

While the attraction pulls in most directly from the nearby suburbs and Philadelphia (just over an hour by car), some even travel to the attraction from other nearby states. One couple I met drove from New York City (over two hours by car), lured in by the claims that the attraction would offer a new level of fear. While the field of disability studies still struggles to gain access to resources in universities and disability activists still have Americans with Disabilities Act compliance denied on the grounds of the expense, this commercial playground of fetishized disability thrives.

And for Pennhurst, the commercialization of its rich history does not start nor stop with the attraction. Pennhurst has enticed several ghost hunter television programs over the years. While these programs typically begin with a description of Pennhurst's history, this backstory is used for the purpose of setting up the drama that then follows, as ghost hunters lock themselves in the building for the night, run around, and report on their findings. Not surprisingly, the crews are always successful at finding the presence of the supernatural, and viewers must take them at their word as they describe the spooky feelings, voices, and sounds they encounter. Here Pennhurst's history is retold in order to help make for good television.[16]

Others believed that Pennhurst would make for a profitable film. Originally due to hit theaters in 2013 but delayed indefinitely, a horror film called *Pennhurst* was on track to add to the genre of haunted asylum films like *Shutter Island*, *Gothika*, *Session 9*, and 2011's *Grave Encounters*, among many others. The setting of an old insane asylum helps set the tone for the *Pennhurst* film, as the plot synopsis describes: "A reality television production crew visits Pennhurst, an abandoned psychiatric hospital, on a mission to capture evidence of paranormal activity. Soon the crew is being picked off one by one in a series of gruesome murders. Turns out there are plenty of ghosts at Pennhurst who don't want the crew there and do everything in their power to make them leave."[17]

Although retitled "*The Lost Episode*," the film was never released commercially. However, the trailer provides another example of people betting on Pennhurst's financial appeal by promoting a version of Pennhurst's history that blurs fiction and fact. Just as the haunted attraction calls upon Bill Baldini's *Suffer the Little Children* exposé, the *Pennhurst* film trailer shows the "reality" television crew watching Baldini's footage on a laptop in one of the old buildings before the attacks begin. While it is not fair to draw conclusions before the film is released, the movie poster suggests that it is extremely unlikely that the film will be more nuanced than Pennhurst's attraction; the lead heroine runs down an abandoned Pennhurst hallway, and we see no villain, just old, rusty wheelchairs and a tagline that reads, *"You'd have to be crazy to go back."*

A more truthful and accurate documentary film (also entitled *Pennhurst*) directed by filmmaker Jodie Alexandra Taylor was released in the summer of 2019 to enthusiastic audiences. Complete with extensive interviews with former residents, Taylor's documentary stands in stark contrast to the paranormal and exploitative genre.[18] Pennhurst provides a vivid example of how the history of institutionalization has been simultaneously forgotten and yet replayed over and over for commercial gain. But Pennhurst should not be seen in isolation. In fact, many other sites across the United States have unleashed the commercial power of the "historic" asylum.

Asylum 49 Haunted Hospital in Tooele, Utah, provides one example. Opened in 1913 as a county poorhouse, it became a hospital out of necessity, though it was severely underfunded. When Kimm Anderson was looking for a site to host a haunted attraction, the location stood out because of its history, now promoted on Asylum 49's website to entice attendees with the question, *"How many people have actually died at the haunted house you're going to?"* (Asylum 49, 2015). Even odder, the building that hosts the Asylum 49 attraction also doubles as a functioning nursing home, yet this does not stop the attraction from pulling in attendees each Halloween, seeking the chance to be scared by actors in straitjackets.

The Trans-Allegheny Lunatic Asylum[19] in Weston, West Virginia, pulls in similar attention each Halloween. Although not the home to a haunted house, attendees can pay to be locked inside for the night. Much like Pennhurst, many people with disabilities were neglected and mistreated here, but now this serves as the site's allure. A 2009 television program on the Travel Channel provided seven hours of live coverage from Trans-Allegheny on Halloween, calling upon the same sensationalized use of history to make for captivating television: "It's a place with a deep and dark history, there was a lot of suffering inside, mentally ill patients were restrained in seclusion cells, lobotomized, some were even murdered, but is this place really haunted? That's what we're about to find out." History makes these Halloween playgrounds marketable.[20]

Locations like Pennhurst provide a gold mine for haunted house entrepreneurs, but using an actual abandoned institution is not easy. In addition to finding one of the sites that has not been torn down or repurposed, creating an attraction like Pennhurst requires a large investment to bring the building up to code. These challenges have not stopped others from capitalizing on the asylum theme simply by creating a fake backstory that claims an asylum once existed at the location. Such haunted houses predate those like Pennhurst and are much more numerous.

A popular haunted attraction in Denver continually ranks as one of the top fright-sites in the country. The backstory explains: "Within the walls of the legendary Nightmare Factory, a hidden passage was unearthed! This passage descended two levels into Gordon Cottingham's Hospital for the Mentally Insane, The Asylum. Much deeper and darker than the previous levels, the Asylum is a damp and musty place infested with spiders, rats, snakes and the endless screams of the tortured souls." Once inside, patients in restraints and muzzles alongside evil doctors and nurses lurk at every corner, but the PR material makes the threat clear: *"Things have gotten out of control at the local insane asylum. The inmates are now running the show."*[21]

The creators of Las Vegas's most popular haunted attraction, "Asylum," explain that their strategy of developing a unified theme was key in standing out from the competition. *Hauntworld Magazine* summarizes their strategy after talking to the entrepreneurs: "You might get startled walking from clown room to vampire room to zombies to aliens, but fear is never really instilled. Jan and Rich believe to do that, they must immerse people in what appears to be a real setting, reinforce the reality, and then devise the fear from that reality!" In fact, when they wanted to expand and create a second attraction that would come to be known as "Hotel Fear," they still made sure to tie in the asylum theme: a patient thought to have been cured by treatment within the asylum returns to the hotel and kills everyone. Like the other haunted attractions tapping into an "asylum" theme, attendees will repeatedly encounter menacing representations of people with mental illness, ready to attack.

In Flint, Michigan, Saint Lucifer's Asylum for the Mentally Insane offers a fictional backstory that takes the details to another level. The attraction's official YouTube trailer begins: "Long ago it was boarded up, abandoned, left for dead, St. Lucifer's Asylum for the Mentally Insane. Once there were over 12,000 patients and a staff of 700, a cutting edge psychiatric hospital specializing in electric shock therapy, but things were far from normal. Patients frequently chewing their tongues off, body counts unusually high. Many patients disappearing in the 5 miles of underground tunnels. . . . Then the state ordered it closed in 1974."[22]

To those familiar with the history of institutions such as Pennhurst, this story sounds perfectly believable, even though the "St. Lucifer" name hints that this history is constructed. Inside the attraction, patients are both the victims of brutal attacks from doctors and nurses and also the harassers of attendees. A particularly upsetting image from the attraction is of a female body that hangs upside down from the ceiling of a shower, covered in blood but stripped down to her bra and underwear. It is not just the general history of institutionalization but also of the most horrific atrocities—the frequent sexual assault of patients—that this attraction appropriates in the pursuit of amusement.

It is hard to say which is more disrespectful: drawing upon the real history of an abandoned institution to help make a thrilling haunted attraction, or completely co-opting history to make an unexciting location seem more exciting. Together, they suggest that the haunting industry, filled with sex, violence, and history, sells. Successfully pulling together all three of these elements, asylums make for good haunted houses that satisfy thrill seekers and entrepreneurs alike. The attraction's commercial success has come at the expense of historical accuracy and the perpetuation of a false narrative that further stigmatizes the former residents.

And in the case of Pennhurst Asylum, it all boiled down to money, helping Chakejian overcome his opponents. Many in the county supported the attraction because it promised job creation in a time of need. As James Conroy, copresident of PMPA, explained to me during the attraction's first year, "Money talks in Chester County, and I don't think we can stop it. . . . He's going to make two million bucks this year, so we have to work out another way . . . to preserve the memory."[23] Chakejian argued that in addition to job creation, the money the attraction brings in would help preserve the site. In fact, he did claim that he poured $2 million into making the attraction safe and up to code. However, making a building safe for a haunted house is quite different from historical preservation, and if the history is lost in the process, what is left to preserve?

Given the clear commercial potential in Pennhurst and other haunted attractions like it, we must question why this theme is so lucrative. Entrepreneurs repeat variations of the same statement to explain it—*"The fear is real!"*—which also became Pennhurst Asylum's catchphrase. But surely, there is more to what appeals here. Without comparing atrocities that are distinct in their own right, would anyone tolerate a haunted attraction physically located at Auschwitz or Ground Zero? If you buy into the claim that Pennhurst is a home for "tortured souls," then the sites of other historic atrocities are likely to be haunted as well. However, it seems safe to assume that these other attractions would not be commercially viable.

That Pennhurst and other haunted asylums draw in such large crowds indicates the lack of historical memory of the injustices committed during the 150 years in which citizens with intellectual and developmental disabilities were isolated, segregated, sterilized, overcrowded, neglected, and abused. The Pennhurst Asylum succeeds because the history is enticing without hitting too close to home for attendees, who are unlikely to understand exactly what happened at

Pennhurst. And because of the haunted attraction's erasure of Pennhurst's real story, even as this history is displayed front and center, it pushes us further away from a future in which the asylum theme would not succeed out of respect for those who once resided in these sites of abuse. For now, people with disabilities are still the source of fear for people across the country each Halloween, an unfortunate reminder of the struggle ahead for disability justice.

When Pennhurst Asylum opened, *Hauntworld* magazine listed it as the scariest haunted attraction in the United States (on a list that also included Denver's Asylum). Since its first year in operation in 2010, Pennhurst Asylum has expanded and reopened annually, adding three new attractions, including the "Dungeon of Lost Souls" where patients were subject to medical experimentation, another historically grounded reality for people with disabilities within institutions.[24]

Shortly after the attraction opened, James Conroy expressed a lack of hope that they could continue to fight the attraction—it was just too popular and too profitable. But additional information about the investors now gives the Pennhurst Memorial and Preservation Alliance cause for hope. The major investors, Mr. Timothy Smith and his son Timothy, have bought out Mr. Chakejian's interest in Pennhurst. Now the sole owners, Mr. Smith and his son want to develop year-round tours on the property, devoting one to the paranormal alongside a second focused on the site's history. They have assured PMPA that the themes would be distinct. According to Conroy, the Smiths have been far more open to feedback from the disability advocacy community, and have expressed a desire that any future tours be respectful and historically accurate. Yet in spite of these conversations, in Halloween 2014, Pennhurst Asylum once again attracted big crowds with its asylum theme. The Smiths' defense? Randy Bates, the experienced haunt entrepreneur hired by Mr. Chakejian to develop the attraction, reportedly held a contract that gave him creative control over Pennhurst Asylum.

Commercialized to an extreme, Pennhurst feels like a twisted incarnation of Disneyland. In the opening weeks of the attraction in 2010, thrill seekers waited for up to four hours in line, paying $25 for admission or $50 for a VIP pass that bought a shortcut to the front of the line. In its first year, it pulled in forty thousand visitors and created traffic jams in the local community. One beverage company even used the crowds to piggyback on Pennhurst's financial success and promoted their new drink with free samples. By 2017, tour prices had escalated to $75 per package, bringing in over $2,000,000 that season alone.[25]

Time will tell whether PMPA's rejuvenated optimism is called for, whether the Smiths will reach out to PMPA leaders to include a voice at the table for people like Jean Searle (a former institutionalized person with a developmental disability), and whether it will even be possible to have a paranormal tour on the grounds that maintains respect for the site's history. As has been echoed on protest signs of many Spring City residents' lawns, we need to use Pennhurst as a site for motivating and promoting "Respect, Not Fear." While Conroy reminds us that "[the story of Pennhurst] has a happy ending. . . . We got them out of Pennhurst, into the community, and they are doing great. Pennhurst proved that there's a better way," he calls the current imagery that makes people with disabilities the objects of fear and horror "the final insult, the final indignity."

## Notes

1. Patrick Walters, "Mental Health Pros Boo Haunted House at Pa. Asylum," *Associated Press*, September 26, 2010, http://opacity.us/article131_mental_health_pros_boo_haunted_house_at_pa_asylum.htm.

2. Anthony Wood, "In Chester County, Suit Seeks to Stop 'Pennhurst Asylum,'" *Philadelphia Inquirer*, September 22, 2010, l. https://www.inquirer.com/philly/news/local/20100922_In_Chester_County__suit_seeks_to_stop__Pennhurst_Asylum_.html.

3. Anthony Wood, "Last Minute Injunction Request Seeks to Halt Friday Opening of Pennhurst Center Haunted House," *Philadelphia Inquirer*, September 24, 2010, https://www.inquirer.com/philly/news/local/20100924_Last-minute_injunction_request_seeks_to_halt_Friday_opening_of_Pennhurst_Center_haunted_house.html.

4. Anthony Wood, "Down to the Wire over Pennhurst," *Philadelphia Inquirer*, September 24, 2010.

5. Randy Bates, "Pennhurst Asylum: America's Scariest Haunted Attraction," *Haunt World Magazine* (2010), https://www.hauntworld.com/featured-article/haunted-house-in-philadelphia-pennsylvania-pennhurst-asylum.

6. All observations regarding the inside of Pennhurst Asylum obtained via ethnographic research by the author during the asylum's first year in operation, October 2010.

7. Bill Baldini has heard this use of the dentist chair since he began reporting on Pennhurst in 1968.

8. Wood, "Down to the Wire."

9. *The Blair Witch Project* was a 1999 horror movie and box office sensation that portrayed three college students lost in the woods of Maryland and menaced by an unknown stalker. The film grossed over $250 million dollars on a shoestring production. It created its own genre and sparked two less successful movies.

10. Walters, "Mental Health Pros Boo Haunted House."

11. "Patients" is terminology used by Mr. Bates that is long outmoded and insensitive. It implies that people with intellectual and developmental disabilities are "sick" and fosters the antiquated, pernicious, and outmoded "medical model" of supporting people with such disabilities. Language in the modern world requires "people first" phrasing, as in "people with disabilities" and "people who lived at Pennhurst."

12. Bates, "Pennhust Asylum."

13. Judith Richardson, *Possession: The History and Uses of Haunting in the Hudson Valley* (Cambridge: Harvard University Press, 2003).

14. Dayle DeLancey, "'How Could It Not Be Haunted': The Haunted Hospital as Historical Record and Ethics Referendum," *Atrium* 6 (2009): 1.

15. "Ticket Prices," Pennhurst Asylum, https://pennhurstasylum.com/tickets.

16. Shows with paranormal themes filmed at Pennhurst thus far include the Travel Channel's *Ghost Adventures* (three times), the SyFy Channel's *Ghost Hunters*, the History Channel, the Discovery Channel's *Destination America*, NBC Peacock Productions, and a seance event filmed by Redrum Productions.

17. Horror News Network (2013). Pennhurst interview with Amanda Dunn, *Horror Movie News*, at https://www.horrornewsnetwork.net/pennhurst-interview-with-amanda-dunn.

18. See http://edu.passionriver.com/pennhurst-documentary.html.

19. This name was changed to Weston State Hospital in 1913, but the original name was resurrected by the owners, presumably for its shock value.

20. Institutions for the mentally and physically disabled are not the only sites where history gets co-opted at Halloween. Each year, thrill seekers in Ohio can visit the "Prison of the Evil Dead" at what was once the Ohio State Reformatory; in Pennsylvania, "Terror Behind the Walls" at the Eastern State Penitentiary; and in West Virginia, "The Dungeon of Horrors" at the West Virginia State Penitentiary. Much like Pennhurst, these prisons met their end as human rights calls for justice brought new standards for how people could be treated. However, on Halloween, the complex reasons for shutting down institutions get superseded by the story, where walls were meant only to keep the dangerous among themselves, rather than to hide abuses from the public.

21. "Asylum 49," Asylum 49: Haunted Hospital and Ghost Tour, http://asylum49.com.

22. "Mini Saint Lucifer's Haunted Asylum Ad," YouTube, http://www.youtube.com/watch?v=OlLde429wsc.

23. James W. Conroy, interview with the author, May 12, 2011.

24. David Rothman and Sheila Rothman, *The Willowbrook Wars: Bringing the Mentally Disabled into the Community* (New Brunswick, N.J.: Harper & Row, 1984); Allen M. Hornblum, Judith L. Newman, and Gregory Dober, *Against Their Will: The Secret History of Medical Experimentation on Children in Cold War America* (New York: Palgrave Macmillan, 2013).

25. "Pennhust Haunted Asylum," https://www.yelp.com/biz/pennhurst-haunted-asylum-spring-city; "Pennhust Asylum," https://pennhurstasylum.com.

# Conclusion

DENNIS B. DOWNEY AND JAMES W. CONROY

Left by his mother in the hands of professionals who assured her that institutionalization was the best option for her son, Roland Johnson (d. 1994) emerged from Pennhurst to become a leading voice for self-advocacy in the disability civil rights movement. Once the victim of assault and abuse, he later was feted by presidents as a role model for his forceful example. To Debbie Robinson and others in the advocacy movement, he often posed the question: "Who's in charge?" Their answer: "We are!"[1]

Shaped by the lived experience of life in an institution, Roland Johnson wrote compassionately in his autobiography, "We're all in this together, and we have to help each other. I think we can learn from each other, and I think the professionals can learn something from us." His was a fitting judgment on the social attitudes and failed policies represented at Pennhurst and other institutions across the country.

Originally known as the Eastern Pennsylvania State Institution for the Feeble-Minded and Epileptic, Pennhurst casts a long shadow over history and the human experience. A model American institution turned nightmare, Pennhurst now holds out the possibility of being a sign of hope. Receding public memory of the horrors that occurred at institutions like Pennhurst, the commercial advantages of site development and the destruction of buildings, and the Pennhurst

Asylum venue and its commercialization of atrocity, all pose substantial obstacles to dignified remembrance.

The most visible sign of hope, however, may be the establishment of a national disability rights museum modeled on the proposed Pennhurst Interpretive Center, but it is only a sign. There is every likelihood a proposed private industrial development will replace the once august physical campus. Already buildings have been demolished and sold for scrap, and souvenir hunters have made off with precious decorative tiles and other valuable objects. The fright-night venue flourishes.

As we trust this volume makes clear, Pennhurst is situated at the epicenter of the disability rights movement, and in many respects it was a catalyst for the social, legal, and policy changes associated with that often-neglected freedom struggle in contemporary America.

As compassion yielded to compliance and coercion, the permanent institutionalization of individuals with intellectual and developmental disabilities (once called the "feeble-minded") was fueled by complex motives. Medical and scientific experts and their political allies were the masterminds—the first perpetrators, if you will. Their vision of creating a world without disabilities (and the "disabled") was pernicious folly and set society on a slippery slope to even greater discrimination, victimization, and human degradation. The numbers are staggering: 10,600 residents at Pennhurst, and over a half million at the more than 250 state institutions erected throughout the twentieth century. (One might also include the more than sixty thousand Americans sterilized by state decree.)

According to a Kennedy administration report, by the early 1960s state governments were spending millions of dollars a year to maintain these facilities for citizens then termed "mentally retarded." That amounts to billions of dollars over the decades simply to warehouse individuals thought to be "unfit" in the struggle for existence. No one has yet tallied the collective human or financial toll for institutions once championed as cost-effective solutions for the "menace of the feeble-minded." Walled off and beyond public view for much of the twentieth century, the conditions could be horrifyingly "grotesque," to use Thurgood Marshall's word. For resident "inmates" and their families, this was the ultimate betrayal of what they had been promised by so-called experts in the field.

Alternatively, the process of deinstitutionalization represents a kind of liberation in one of the most dramatic social transformations of the last half century. Thanks to advocacy and litigation, former residents had basic constitutional protections restored, including a right to live in the community and pursue purposeful lives through public education, employment, and support services. As the path-breaking Pennhurst Longitudinal Study proved, people are better off and society will be enriched if the proper supports are in place. Like *PARC* and *Halderman v. Pennhurst*, the Americans with Disabilities Act (1990), which was strongly influenced by what we learned at Pennhurst, stands as a landmark in civil rights history. Now three decades old, the ADA served as a basis for the sweeping United Nations Convention on the Rights of Persons with Disabilities or CRPD (2007).

But as we said at the outset, this is a cautionary tale in which the current impetus for inclusion and equal rights has been accompanied by new challenges and uncertainties. For example, in 2014 the United States Senate failed to ratify the CRPD treaty on a purely partisan vote. Senate Republicans stood in opposition despite the impassioned plea of World War II veteran Bob Dole, who was severely wounded and left with a physical disability from his combat experience.

Moreover, what Anthony Imparato, Nicholas Kristof, and others have called the "new eugenics"—a reference to new frontiers in bioethics and genetic engineering—has gained a degree of scientific and social acceptance.[2] There are respectable psychologists and ethicists calling for a return to state institutionalization as a more cost-effective alternative to community-based residential placements.[3] They argue that one just needs to avoid the mistakes of the past. The experiences of residents at Pennhurst and elsewhere demonstrate the short-sightedness and lack of historical perspective inherent in such policy recommendations. In the wake of gun violence in El Paso, Dayton, and elsewhere in the summer of 2019, President Donald Trump has championed building new institutions to house the mentally ill.[4]

Among other considerations, advocates point out that it costs nearly twice as many dollars annually to maintain someone in an institution.

From the most recent (2014) national data, the average expenditure (state and federal) for supporting a person in an institution was $194,316; in a community setting the total was as low as $61,710.[5] In Pennsylvania, for example, the cost of institutional placement has increased with the declining population and the Commonwealth's effort to close institutions altogether. At Polk State Center, as it is now called, the costs of maintaining an individual in residence can exceed $400,000 per year.[6]

As we conclude our writing at the end of 2019, what remains of the former Pennhurst State School and Hospital exists in four parts:

1. Old campus—the earliest buildings, now privately owned and dominated by its use as a Halloween amusement.
2. Upper Campus—all but one of the five major structures from the 1930s and later were demolished in mid-2017. This part of Pennhurst was also called the "Women's Campus," because it was intended for segregation based on gender. Neglect of the buildings led to roof and water damage that made them unsalvageable. The one structure remaining houses a National Guard unit in Audubon Hall.
3. New Horizon building—this early 1970s, hospital-like building is now repurposed, ironically, as an institutional residential setting for injured and aged military veterans. It has been extended with recent construction. It is now called the Southeastern Veterans Center, Coates Hall.
4. The superintendent's mansion—the original home of the Pennhurst superintendents from 1908 to 1987 still stands on property currently controlled by the Department of Military and Veterans Affairs.

In the summer of 2017, however, the property's owners began the process of demolishing many of the historic structures. They have been careful not to interfere with the Pennhurst Asylum venue that brings in several million dollars in revenue each autumn. The demolition project itself, intended to make way for a sprawling commercial center, added a new note of uncertainty to the task of preserving the memory of the infamous institution.

The superintendent's mansion had become the focus of efforts to establish a place for respectful memory and an International Site of Conscience for Pennhurst and places like it. The Pennhurst Memorial and Preservation Alliance, in partnership with other regional organizations, has been working to transform this venerable structure into an interpretive center dedicated to representing and educating about the institution's place in American history. To that end, in October 2018 Governor Tom Wolf signed SB 353 permitting the PMPA to purchase the superintendent's mansion. If successful, an interpretive center will provide a dignified memorial, in contrast to the Pennhurst Asylum attraction, which in the past has demeaned and degraded the memory of the 10,600 people who lived and died at the institution. Which will win out—the Asylum venue and commercial park or the memorial site—is an open question.

A decade ago, the Pennhurst Memorial and Preservation Alliance had hoped to help repurpose the Old Campus into new, socially responsible applications—including community centers, condos, day care, and a museum. When the Old Campus was sold and the Halloween attraction began advertising on Facebook to hire local youth to "*play a scary psyco* [*sic*]," that hope evaporated. The group simply could not be associated with "the final indignity" of that use of the property.

The PMPA therefore determined to pursue other ways to tell the crucial American story of the disability rights movement through the lens of Pennhurst. In 2010, a Pennsylvania Historical Marker was installed on the state highway next to the Pennhurst campus. The audience was reportedly larger than any that had ever attended such a marker dedication. A year later a short documentary film was produced entitled *A Call of Conscience* that has been viewed across America. Several years after that, a fuller public television documentary called *I Go Home* presented a fuller picture of life at Pennhurst. A sequal entitled *Going Home* aired in 2019. Jodie Alexandra Taylor's new commercial documentary, which includes interviews with former residents and staff, was released in the summer of 2019 and is being shown on college campuses and small commercial theaters.

On July 25, 2015, hundreds of people gathered at Philadelphia's Independence Mall to commemorate the twenty-fifth anniversary of the signing of the Americans with Disabilities Act, the great civil rights statute that changed America for the better. The symbolic juxtaposition of a speakers' platform on the steps of the National Constitution Center and the Liberty Bell at the opposite end, with a tidal wave of humanity between, provided a fitting stage. People of varying abilities, backgrounds, and life experiences came together to celebrate and to remember. Members of the Pennhurst Memorial and Preservation Alliance helped to organize the Independence Mall event, and for them there was a special meaning in the Philadelphia location, where Pennhurst's story had begun. Like many others, they had dedicated their adult lives to the cause of equality and citizenship regardless of one's station or status.

Beginning in 2015, PMPA sponsored a Traveling Exhibit on Pennhurst and Disability History, as well as the creation of several documentary films. To date, this educational campaign has met with resounding success, including displays and screenings in the Pennsylvania state capitol, dozens of colleges and advocacy organizations, and several foreign countries. The exhibit was placed in the United States Senate Russell office building, accompanied by a panel discussion in the Capitol Visitor's Center (June 27, 2016). Pennsylvania Senator Bob Casey hosted the event, which drew hundreds of people interested in Pennhurst's significance in public health policy. Less than a year later, Senator Casey displayed a photograph of the Pennhurst Administration building in the Senate chamber during the contentious debate over the repeal of the Affordable Care Act ("Obamacare"). The iconic image served as a potent visual reminder of what could go wrong in health care if the most vulnerable are stigmatized and taken advantage of by those meant to protect them.

Furthermore, the juxtaposition of the Pennhurst Asylum Halloween venue and the proposed Pennhurst Museum / Interpretive Center illustrates that the Pennhurst narrative is not yet concluded. One seeks to exploit the former residents through a fabricated and demeaning storyline, and the other seeks their redemption by restoring dignity and honor to those once cast aside. The next steps in letting the public know about one of America's great civil rights movements are ready for implementation. This effort will require substantial fundraising.

In the spring of 2017, Pennhurst's Old Campus and the Asylum haunted house attraction were sold to new owners. Almost immediately, the PMPA began working with current venue management to reduce the pernicious disability imagery in the attraction, and to conceive of joint efforts that will further the goal of public education and understanding about life at Pennhurst. The owner's decision to tear down historic structures and excavate the landscape—to "improve" the property—makes historic preservation efforts all the more urgent. The superintendent's mansion is now in jeopardy and likely will be demolished as a part of the new commercial center that is under development.

The debate over the relative importance of historical memory and commercial profit is being heard across the Commonwealth of Pennsylvania. In Allentown, Wyomissing, and out to rural Venango County north of Pittsburgh, the Commonwealth government has set its sights on closing institutions that cared for individuals with mental illnesses, intellectual disabilities, and other chronic conditions. Proposals to close Norristown and Allentown State Hospitals in the east, the Hamburg and Embreeville Centers in the midstate, and the Polk Center in the west, and move residents to community residential care, had ignited old conflicts over where residents "belong." The Commonwealth's new policy of ending institutional care, which advocates usually support and some families oppose, has also introduced the thorny issue of what to do with vacated buildings and grounds in an era of increasing land values in what are now suburban areas. On each of these points, Pennhurst provides a meaningful and representative example of both prudent and ill-conceived public policy outcomes.

The global struggle for disability rights that Pennhurst helped to shape is really a struggle for *human* rights. Through advocacy, litigation, and courageous perseverance, public disability policy changed and the worst features of eugenics-inspired medical and social engineering gave way to a fuller measure of liberty, equal protection, and dignity. Institutions closed, public facilities were made accessible, and services and supports provided an essential safety net for fellow citizens.

Although social attitudes have begun to change, remnants of the old stereotypes and prejudices regarding disabilities persist. But on balance, Pennhurst and the disability rights movement have enlarged public consciousness about such core constitutional principles as equal protection, due process, and prohibitions against cruel and unusual punishment. Phrases like "self-determination," "reasonable accommodations," "behavioral therapy," and "least restrictive environment" are now part of social discourse and public policy. Given their prevalence in the general population, people are far more aware of Autism Spectrum Disorder, Multiple Disabilities, Down syndrome, and other clinical diagnoses. Suffice it to say, advocacy and litigation tied to conditions at Pennhurst played a crucial role in this process of greater public awareness and understanding.

Bill Baldini could not have known in 1968 that the *Suffer the Little Children* documentary series would ignite a transformation in public attitudes toward people with intellectual disabilities. Beginning in Philadelphia and then rippling across the country, the five-part exposé introduced a new style of investigative journalism. Nor could Baldini have imaged how his work would inspire other journalists, like Geraldo Rivera at Willowbrook, to investigate the underside of institutional incarceration. They put a very human face on nightmarish conditions that were then broadcasted into family living rooms. The power of the media and broadcast journalism cannot be underestimated.

Pennhurst provides an apt example of this human rights movement because in many key ways it became the locus of groundbreaking progress. The first victory in the right to a free appropriate public education was won over the deplorable conditions at Pennhurst (*PARC v. Commonwealth*). The first legal challenge to large-scale segregation in public institutions, not aiming to fix the institutions but to end them, happened because of Pennhurst (*Halderman v. Pennhurst*). And the first hint of a right to decent treatment according to professional standards was won there (*Romeo v. Youngberg*).

The lessons learned at Pennhurst changed America, and they are inspiring global change in disability policy. Large-scale segregation of children, or adults, is counterproductive. Dorothea Dix and Samuel

Gridley Howe understood, and we know this now. Pennhurst was instrumental in this sea change in policy and public awareness.

What America has accomplished in nearly ending its reliance on large public institutions for people with intellectual and developmental disabilities is now the subject of tremendous interest overseas. The global community is eager to learn "how" the Pennhurst exodus, and the deinstitutionalizations that followed, were accomplished with quality and dignity. The Pennhurst story has been told to audiences of students, advocates, and policy makers in more than a dozen nations.[7] Part of a larger narrative of disability history, Pennhurst's story has been inspirational in showing that "there is a better way": investing in inclusive community supports is pragmatically and ethically more humane and productive than further isolation and segregation.

It is difficult to distill all of what has been learned during the past fifty years of American progress toward dignity and rights for citizens with disabilities—but the perspective of the tragedies and triumphs related to Pennhurst does lead to these seven learning points:

1. There is a better way.
2. Human potential is great indeed.
3. There is value in litigation.
4. Relationships and connectedness are at the heart of quality of life.
5. The lessons of Pennhurst are international in scope.
6. Supported self-determination works.
7. The nation needs a place of remembrance.

The urge to remember is a very human trait, and it provides the occasion for informed public policy that regresses history's nightmare moments. Remembrance can also encourage hope in a better future, a sentiment on display during the June 2016 Pennhurst program in the Russell Senate Office Building. Hundreds of people came with walkers and in wheelchairs, with aides and service dogs, and a range of behavioral and cognitive challenges. Some seemed more "typical," but collectively the audience demonstrated the full spectrum of humanity and disability. Legislative staff and disability advocates crowded into the small auditorium. Pennsylvania Senator Robert Casey served as host and offered introductory remarks. It was a hopeful moment in the long struggle for disability rights.

What brought them together was the shared recognition that the Pennhurst experience spoke to history and the present moment, and to the possibilities of a better and more compassionate future. Someone remarked that there was no escaping the fact that disability was part of our common humanity. Mention was made of Betty Potts, Roland Johnson, and the other Pennhurst residents who had left the institution as a result of the great historic freedom struggle now being celebrated. In the sustained applause that greeted Tom Gilhool and other advocates, it seemed possible for a fleeting moment that the anguished history of Pennhurst might be redeemed by what poet Seamus Heaney called the "longed-for tidal wave of justice."

## Notes

1. Roland Johnson quoted in the documentary *I Go Home*, WITF Media, 2016.

2. Nicholas Kristoff, "The New Eugenics," *New York Times*, July 4, 2003, https://www.nytimes.com/2003/07/04/opinion/the-new-eugenics.html; Jack Palmer, "The New Eugenics: Genetic Engineering," http://www.ulm.edu/~palmer/NewEugenics.htm.

3. Dominic A. Sisti, Andrea G. Segal, and Ezekiel J. Emanuel, "Improving Long-Term Psychiatric Care: Bring Back the Asylum," *Journal of the American Medical Association* 313, no. 3 (January 2015): 243–44, http://jamanetwork.com/journals/jama/article-abstract/2091312. The authors' argument extends to populations with mental illness and intellectual and developmental disabilities.

4. See https://www.washingtonpost.com/politics/trump-says-the-us-should-build-more-psychiatric-institutions-in-response-to-rising-gun-violence/2019/08/15/bb9b24e8-bfa5-11e9-9b73-fd3c65ef8f9c_story.html.

5. Medicaid's Intermediate Care Facilities program for People with Developmental Disabilities or ICF; Medicaid's Home and Community Based Services or "Waiver" program; S. A. Larson, H. J. Eschenbacher, L. L. Anderson, B. Taylor, S. Pettingell, A. Hewitt, M. Sowers, and M. L. Fay, *In-Home and Residential Long-Term Supports and Services for Persons with Intellectual or Developmental Disabilities: Status and Trends Through 2014* (Minneapolis: University of Minnesota, Research and Training Center on Community Living, Institute on Community Integration, 2017), available at https://risp.umn.edu/publications.

6. "Pennsylvania Will Close Two State Centers for Intellectually Disabled," https://www.post-gazette.com/news/social-services/2019/08/14/Closure-Polk-State-center-White-Haven-State-intellectually-disabled-venango-luzerne/stories/201908140079.

7. Australia, Belgium, Canada, England, Finland, Georgia Republic, Ireland, Israel, Kosovo, Lithuania, Mexico, Russia, Serbia, Sweden, Trinidad (OAS), Ukraine, and the entire European Union via several talks to the European Association of Service Providers for Persons with Disabilities.

# Gallery

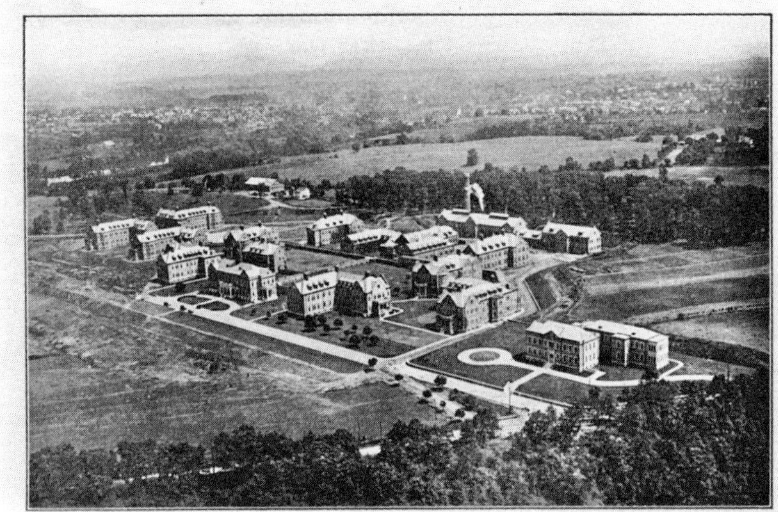


GALLERY 1 Pennhurst campus aerial view, 1922.

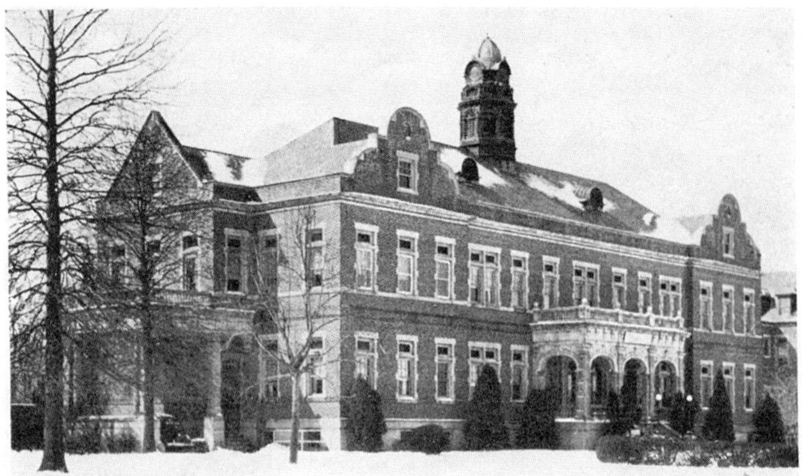

GALLERY 2 Pennhurst administration building, 1920.

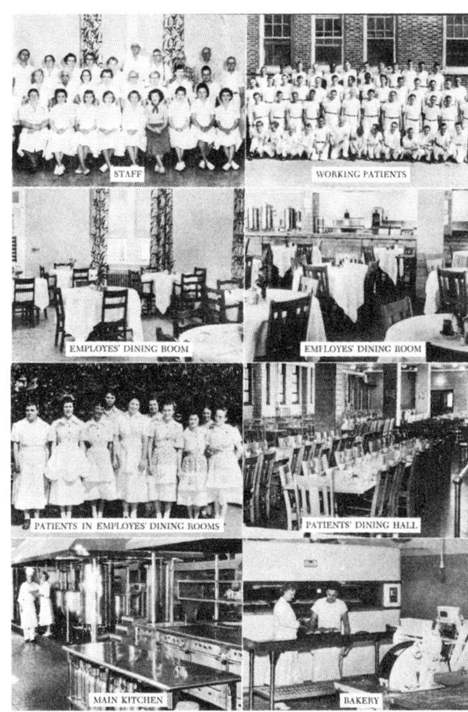


GALLERY 3 Staff and "working patients," 1954.

GALLERY 4 Dining hall segregated by gender, 1916. Note evidence of order under supervision.

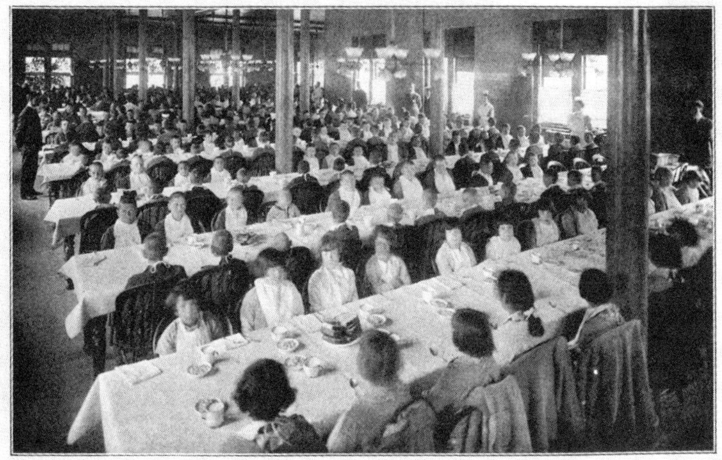

ONE OF THE DINING ROOMS

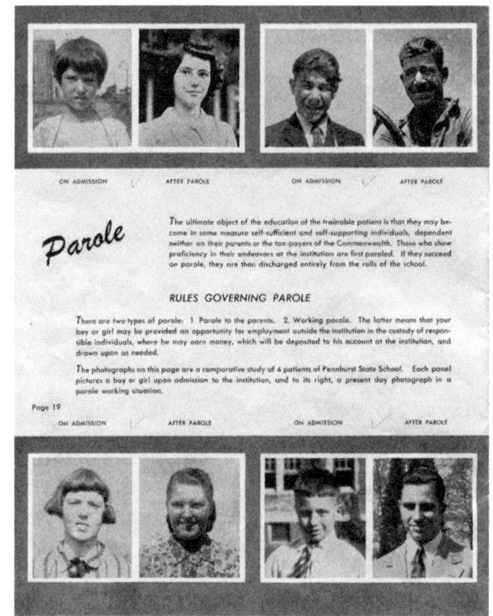

ON ADMISSION AFTER PAROLE ON ADMISSION AFTER PAROLE

*Parole*

The ultimate object of the education of the trainable patient is that they may become in some measure self-sufficient and self-supporting individuals, dependent neither on their parents or the tax-payers of the Commonwealth. Those who show proficiency in their endeavors at the institution are first paroled. If they succeed on parole, they are then discharged entirely from the rolls of the school.

RULES GOVERNING PAROLE

There are two types of parole: 1 Parole to the parents. 2. Working parole. The latter means that your boy or girl may be provided an opportunity for employment outside the institution in the custody of responsible individuals, where he may earn money, which will be deposited to his account at the institution, and drawn upon as needed.

The photographs on this page are a comparative study of 4 patients of Pennhurst State School. Each panel pictures a boy or girl upon admission to the institution, and to its right, a present day photograph in a parole working situation.

Page 19

ON ADMISSION AFTER PAROLE ON ADMISSION AFTER PAROLE

GALLERY 5 Rules governing parole—trial releases prior to discharge—before and after photos, ca. 1940.

GALLERY 6 Toilets lacking privacy. Photo taken ca. 1970 as a demonstration.

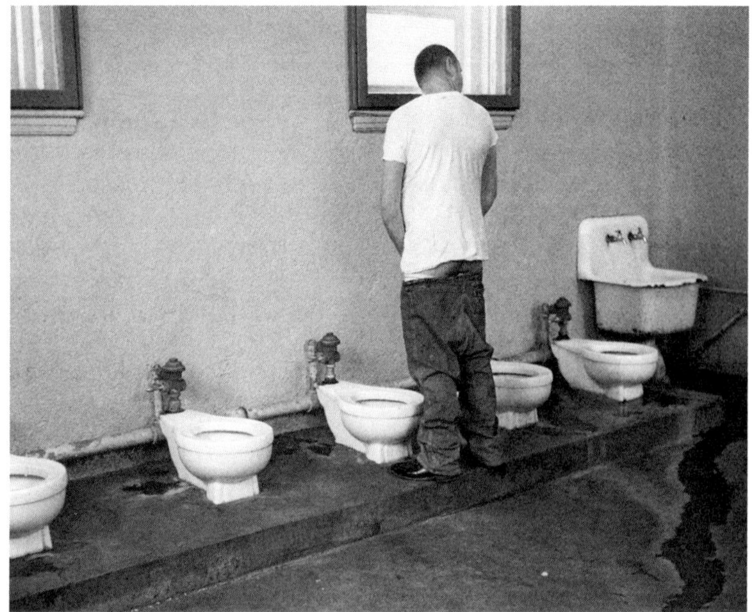

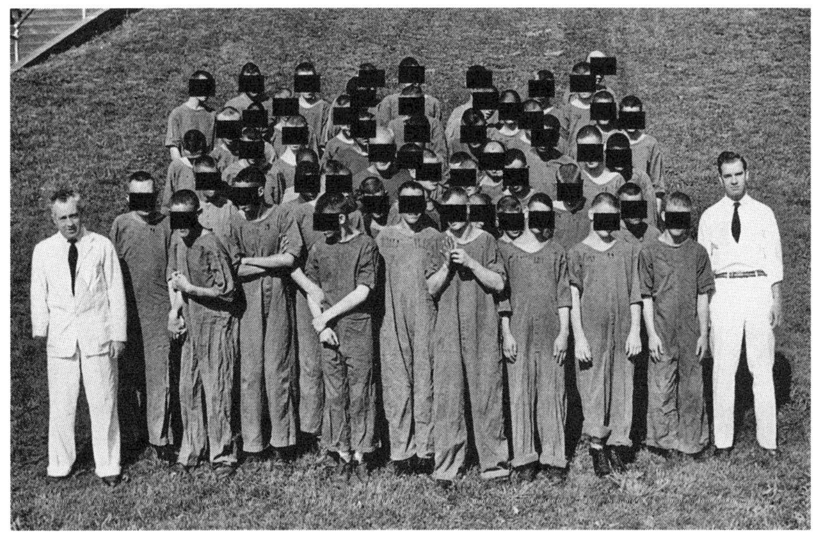

GALLERY 7 Young men in uniform dress and haircuts, interracial, ca. 1960.

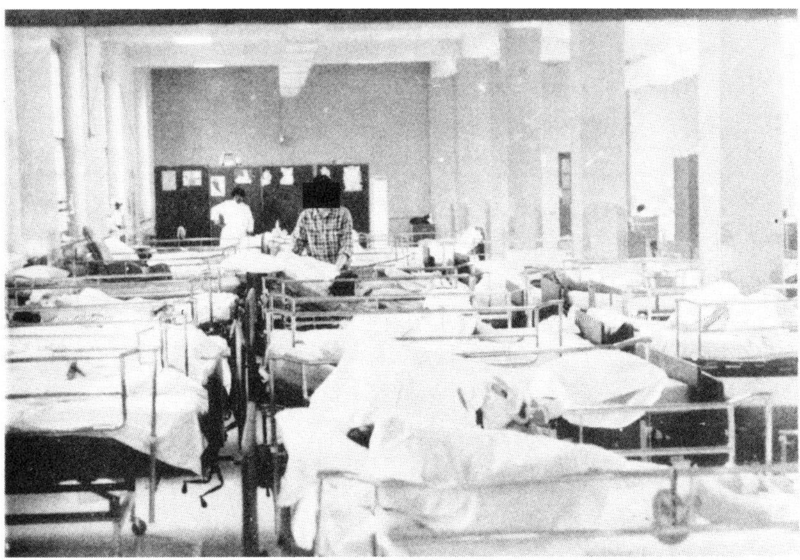

GALLERY 8 Crowded beds at Pennhurst. Photo taken by FBI in 1975.

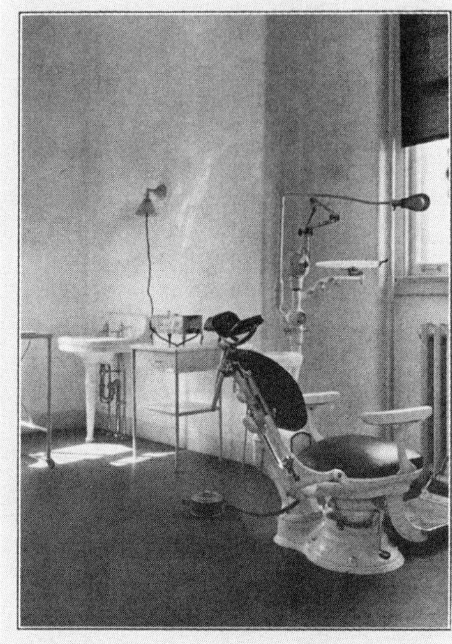


GALLERY 9 Dental surgery clinic, ca. 1925.

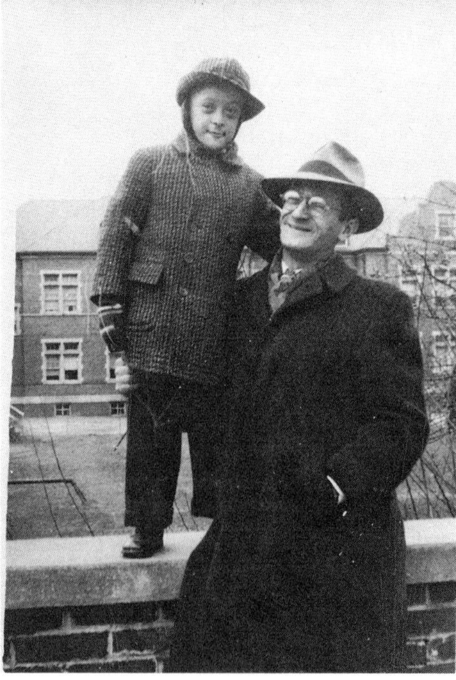

GALLERY 10 Albert New with his son Martin upon admission in 1944.

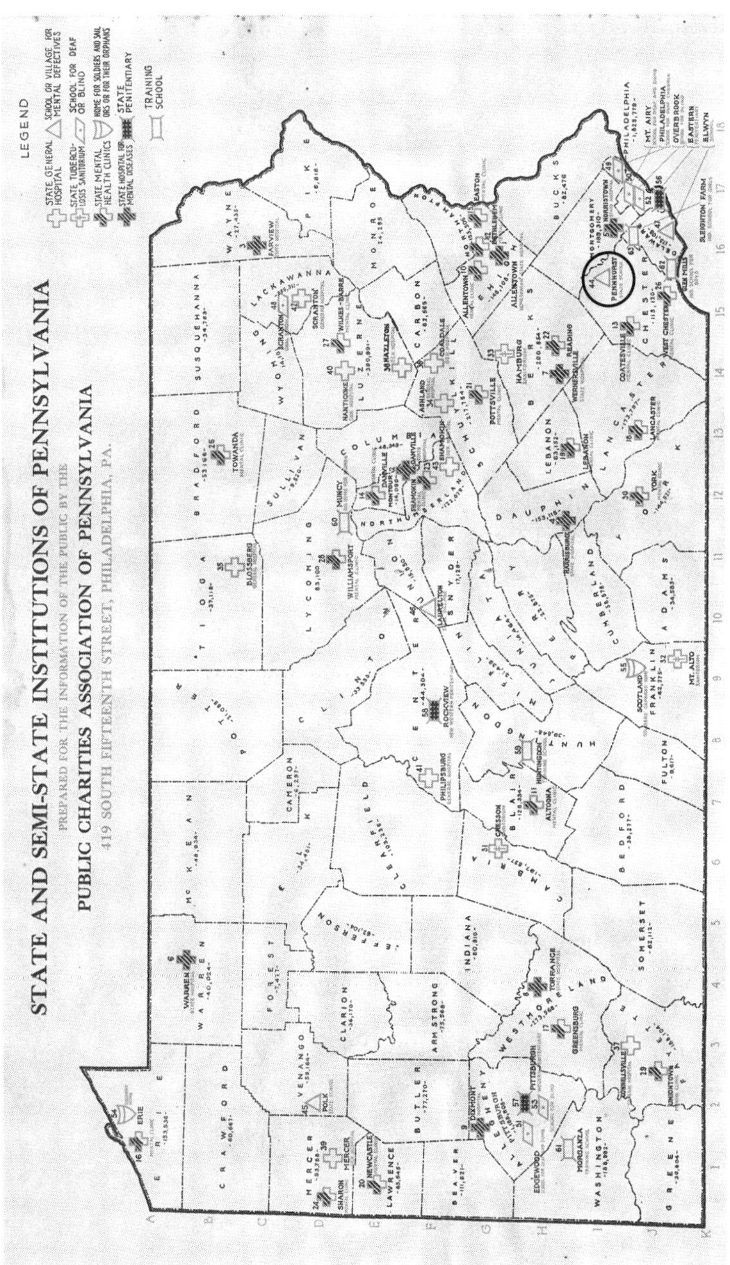


GALLERY 11 Pennsylvania map of institutions, ca. 1923.

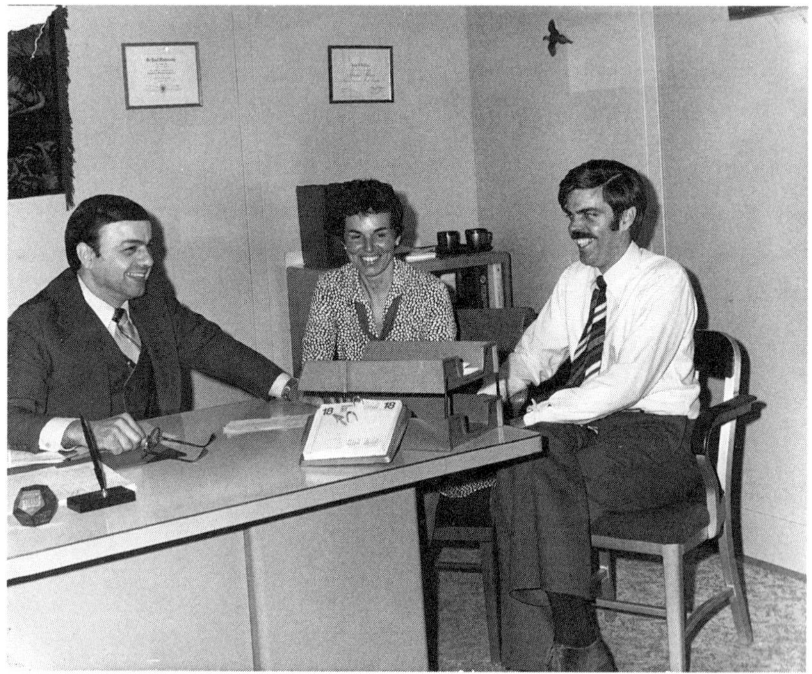

GALLERY 12 Key actors in *Halderman v. Pennhurst*: Peter Polloni, Arc director then state agency director; Carla Morgan, special master for the court; Tom Gilhool, lead attorney for the Arc of Pennsylvania.

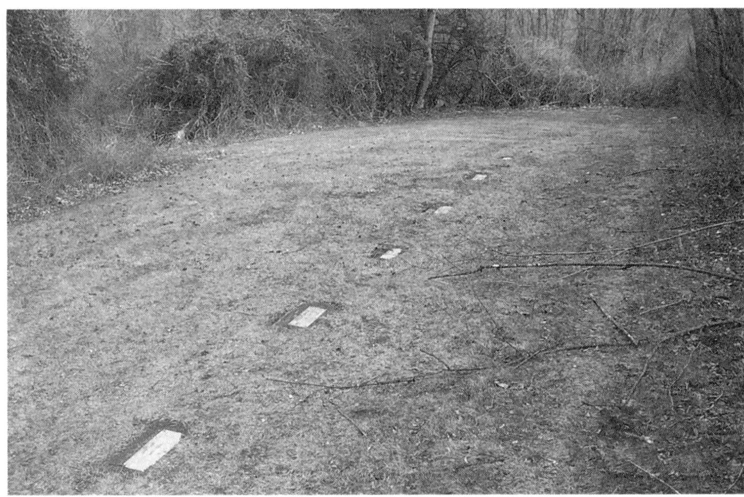

GALLERY 13 Some of the forty marker stones at the Pennhurst Cemetery, nearly all from the 1918 epidemic of Spanish flu.

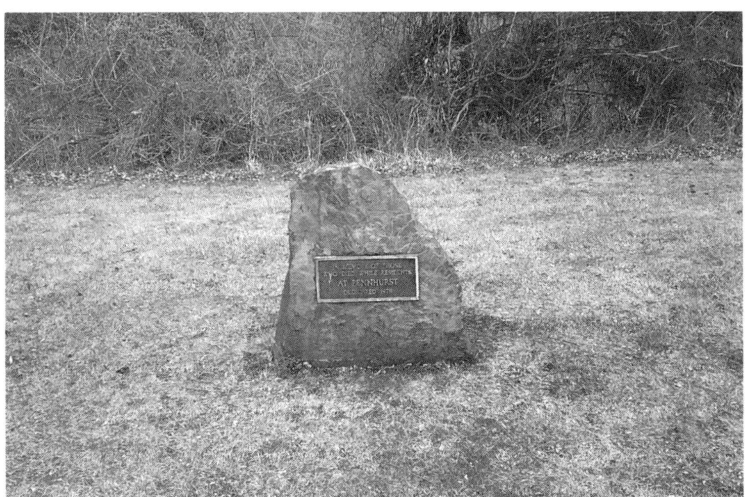


GALLERY 14 Stone commemorating conversion of marker stones from numbers to names, 1978.

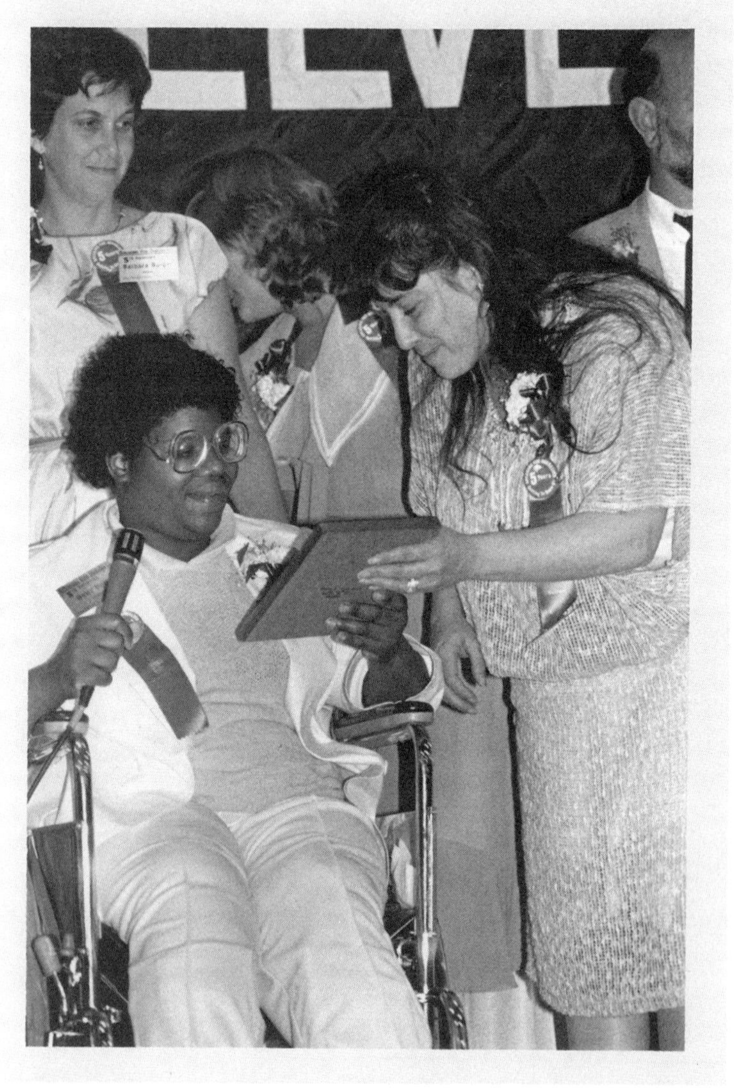

GALLERY 15 Elizabeth "Betty" Potts, first person to leave Pennhurst under Judge Broderick's federal court order, accepting award at Speaking for Ourselves Banquet, 1987.

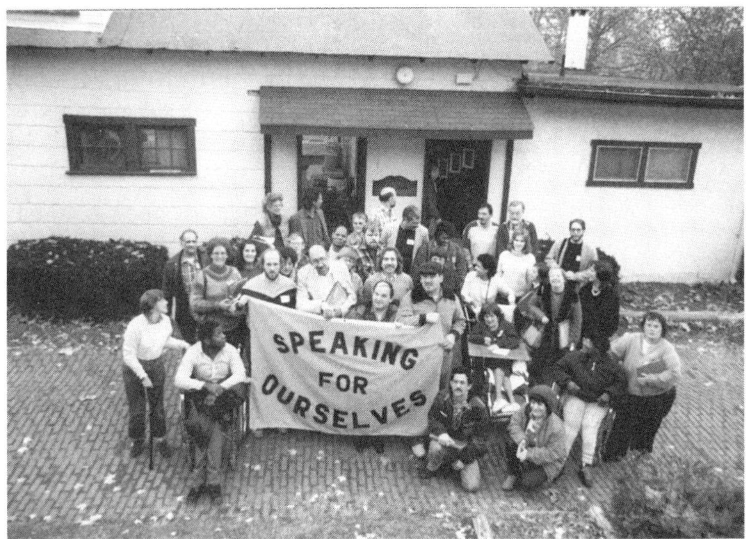


GALLERY 16 Speaking for Ourselves Retreat at Fellowship Farm, 1987.

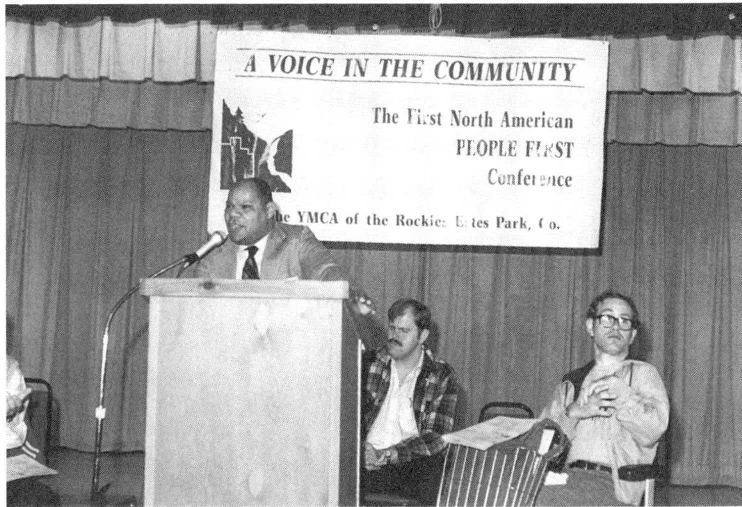


GALLERY 17 Speaking for Ourselves president Roland Johnson at the First North American People First Conference, 1990.

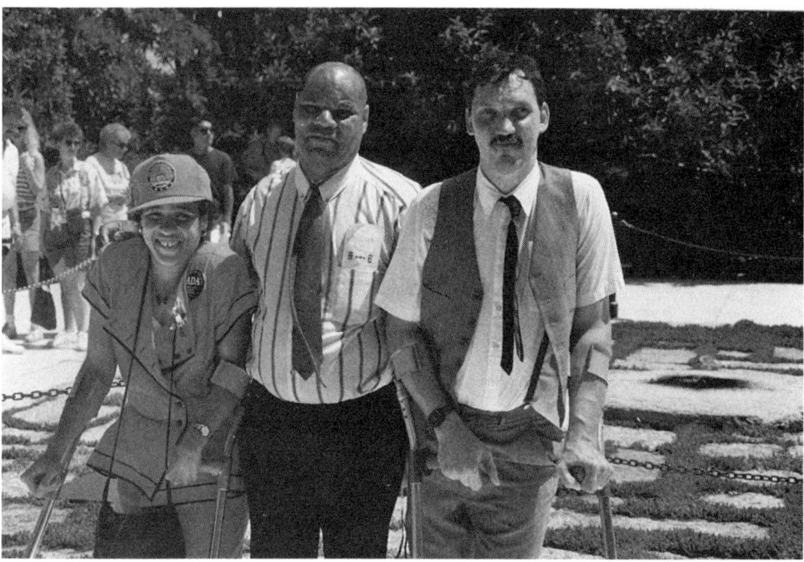

GALLERY 18 Speaking for Ourselves officers Debbie Robinson, Roland Johnson, and Steve Dorsey at the White House ADA signing, 1990.

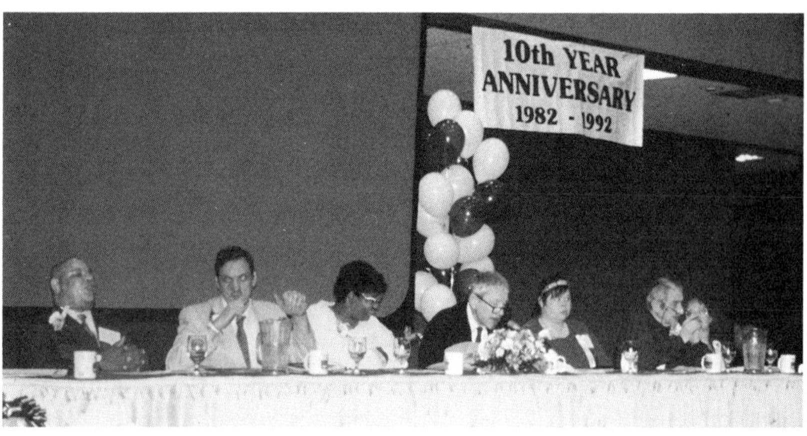


GALLERY 19 Speaking for Ourselves Tenth Anniversary Banquet, 1992—Roland Johnson, Steve Dorsey, Betty Potts, Justin Dart, Luann Carter, Gunnar Dybwad.

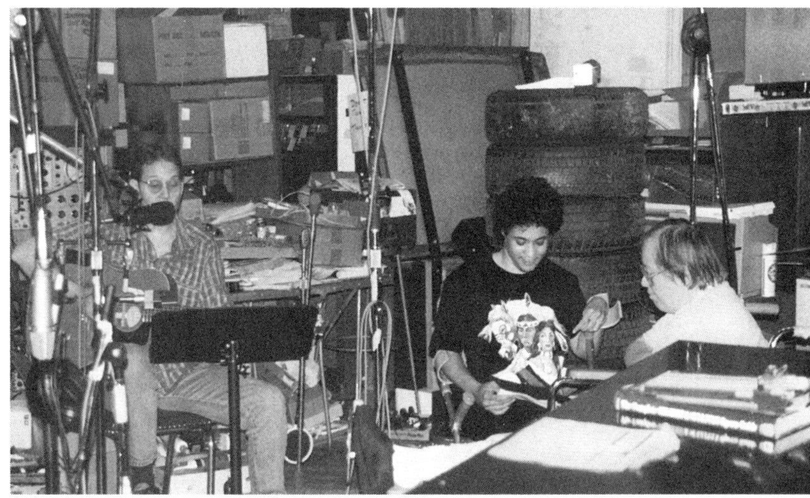

GALLERY 20 Recording the Speaking for Ourselves anthem with Karl Williams, Debbie Robinson, and Luann Carter, 1995.

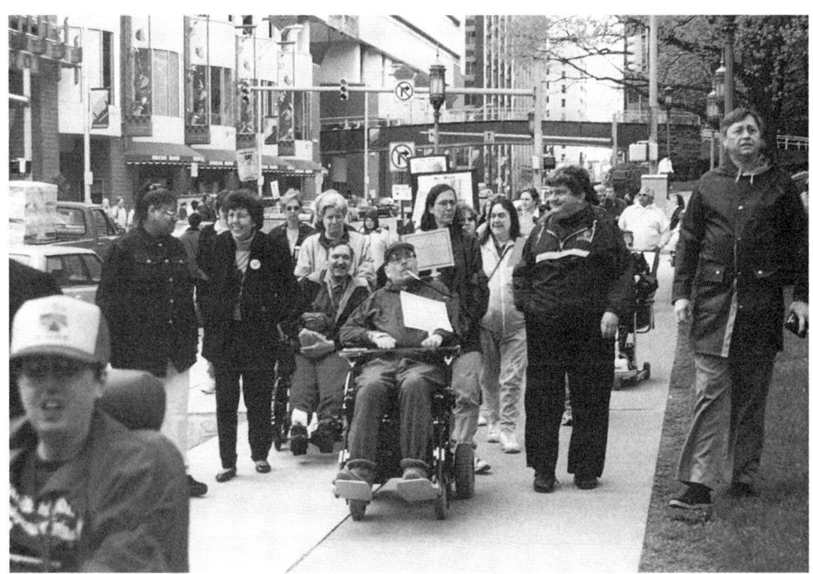

GALLERY 21 March to the Capitol to close institutions, 2000.

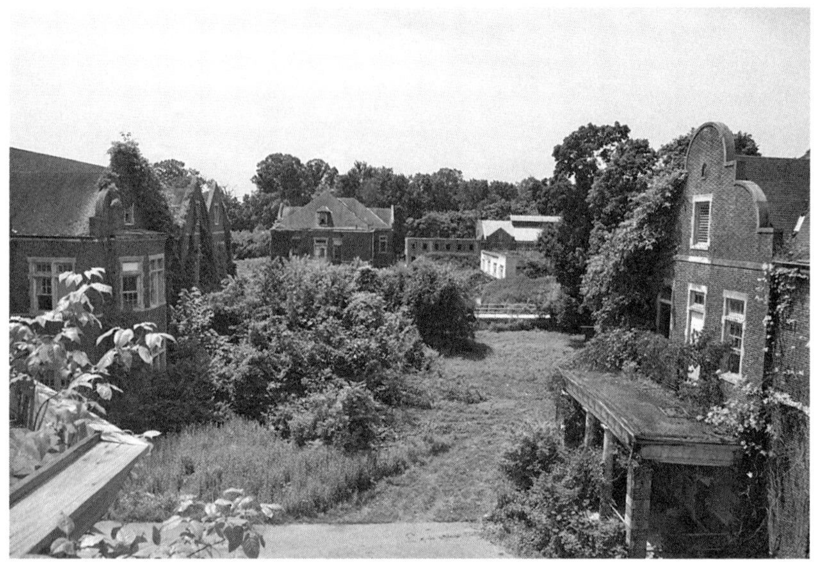

GALLERY 22 The decay of Pennhurst courtyard from 1987 to 2007.

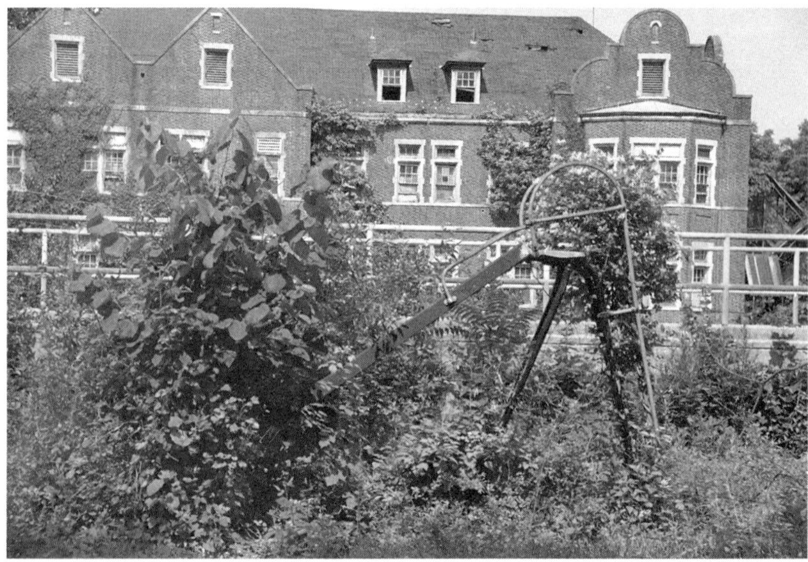

GALLERY 23 Decay of Devon Hall with adjacent playground, 2007.

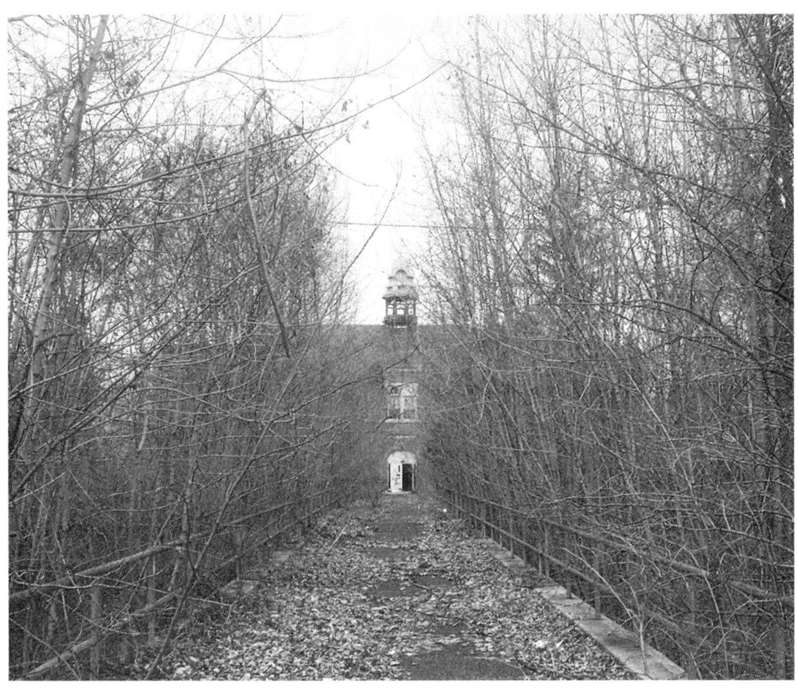

GALLERY 24 Decay shown by overgrowth at approach to the administration building, 2008.

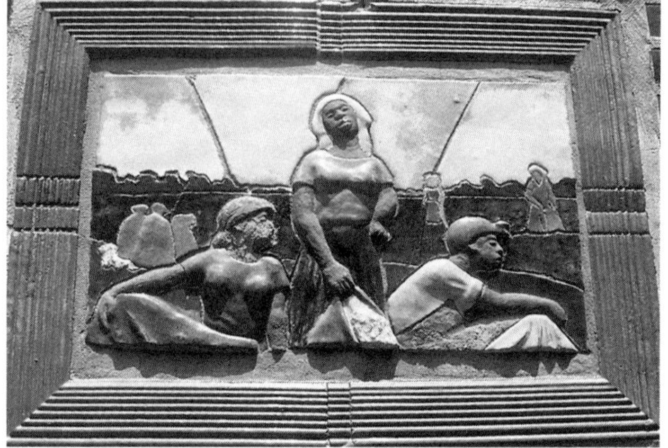

GALLERY 25 Original decorative art on administration building prior to decay.

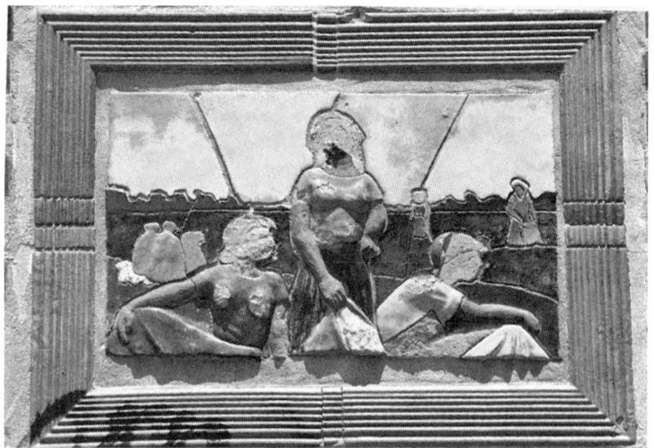

GALLERY 26 Defaced decorative art, 2014.

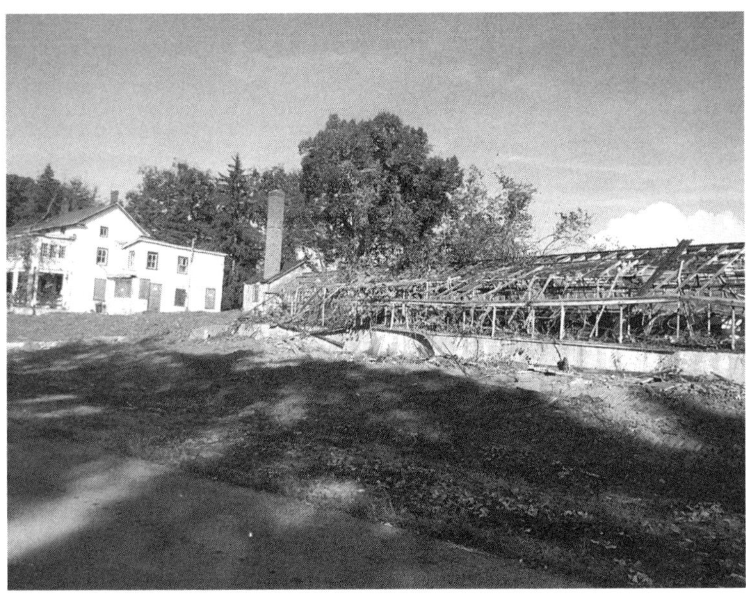

GALLERY 27 Physician's mansion and greenhouse in decay prior to demolition, 2016.

9 —The Towers property purchased for the State Hospital.
E. D. Miller, Publisher—Parkerford, Pa.

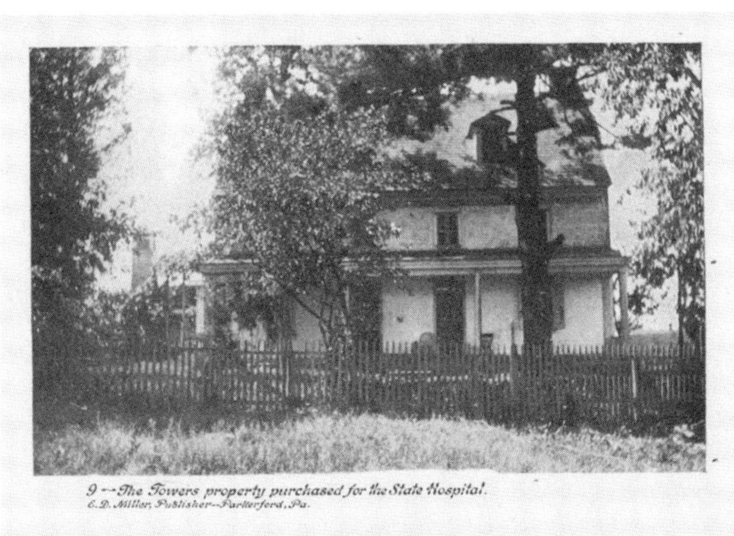

GALLERY 28 Original appearance of physician's mansion, ca. 1920.

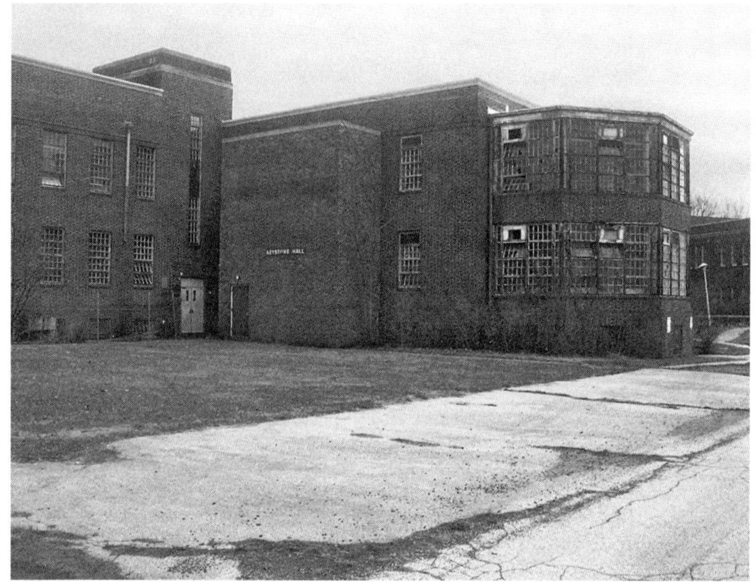

GALLERY 29 Keystone Hall with glass block dayrooms, prior to demolition, 2008.

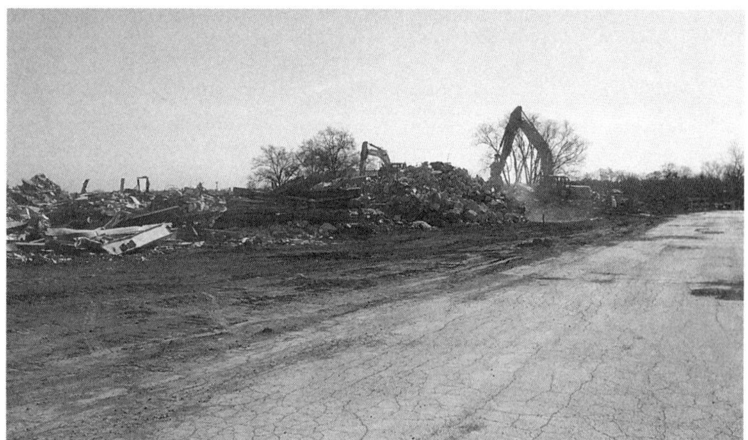

GALLERY 30 Keystone Hall remains after demolition, 2017.

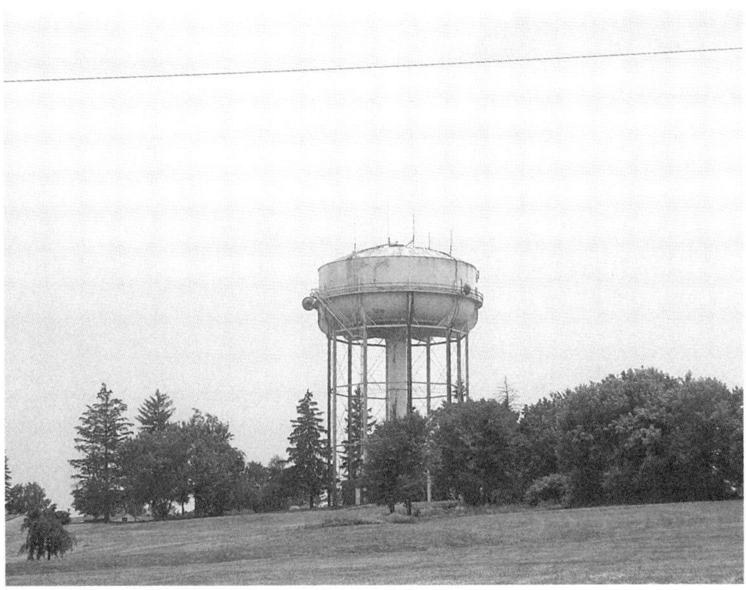

GALLERY 31 Pennhurst water tower, a local landmark for decades, 2006.

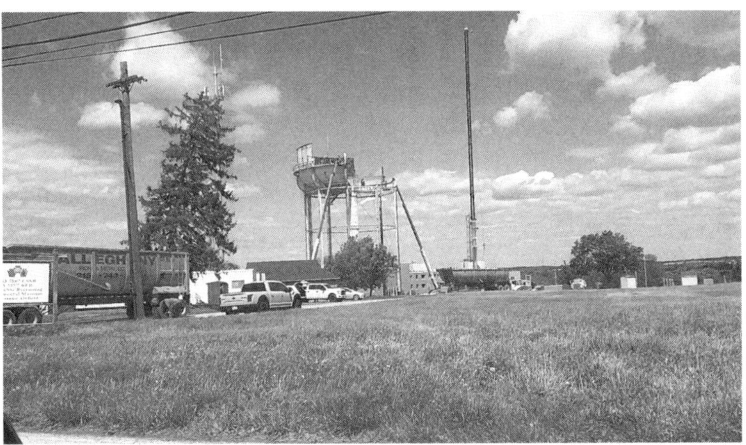

GALLERY 32 Water tower in the midst of demolition, 2017.

PENNHURST STATE
SCHOOL & HOSPITAL
Between 1908 and 1987, more than 10,500 Pennsylvanians with developmental disabilities lived here. Public controversy over the inhumane treatment of residents and two decades of complex litigation, including three arguments before the US Supreme Court, led to the institution's closure. Groundbreaking advocacy and new public policy, including transition to community-based living, made Pennhurst a milestone in the disabilities civil rights movement.

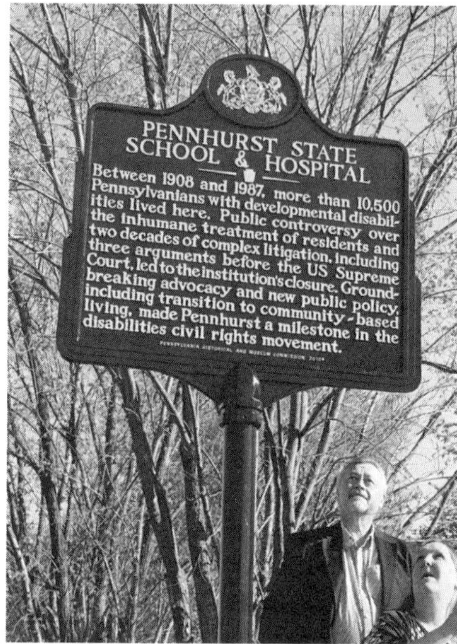

GALLERY 33 Pennhurst marker dedication, 2010.

GALLERY 34 Superintendent's mansion, to be preserved to commemorate the Pennhurst history.

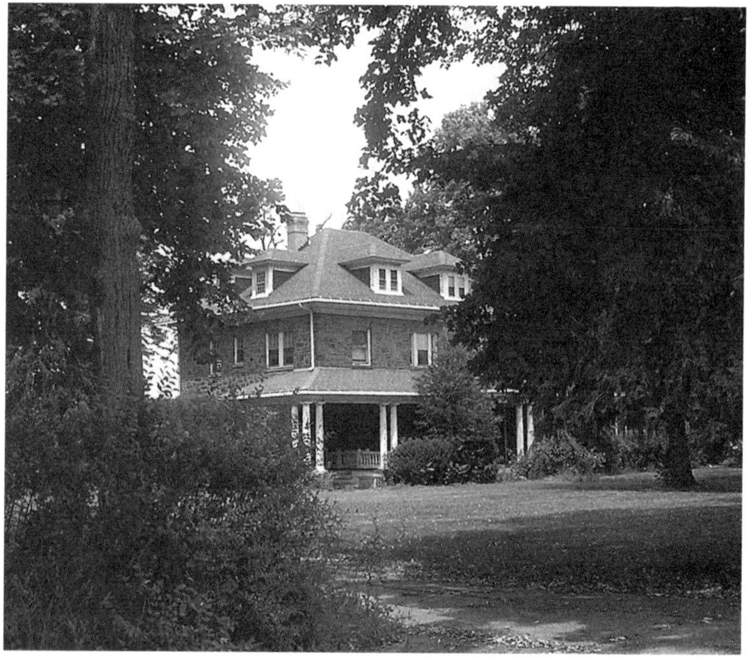

## *Timeline of Pennhurst State School and Hospital*

For a more detailed timeline, see "Pennhurst Timeline," Pennhurst Memorial and Preservation Alliance, http://preservepennhurst.org/default.aspx?pg=93.

1852 Privately operated Pennsylvania Training School for Idiotic and Feeble-Minded Children opens in Germantown; cornerstone for new school and farm laid in 1856 at Elwyn near Media, Delaware County.

1876 During Centennial Exhibition, Elwyn hosts inaugural meeting of Association of Medical Officers of American Institutions for Idiotic and Feeble-Minded Persons (now AAIDD).

1893 Commonwealth of Pennsylvania authorizes State Institution for the Feeble-minded of Western Pennsylvania at Polk in Venango County; opens 1897.

1903 Commonwealth authorizes Eastern Pennsylvania State Institution for the Feebleminded and Epileptic (Pennhurst).

1905 Gov. Samuel Pennypacker vetoes sterilization bill; proponents undeterred.

1906 Dr. H. H. Goddard leaves West Chester Normal School to direct Vineland (N.J.) Training School; 1912 publishes *The Kallikak Family*.

1908 Pennhurst opens on Crab Hill near Spring City, Chester County; Charles H. Frazier, MD, authors *The Menace of the Feebleminded in Pennsylvania*.

1911 Commonwealth and Philadelphia Department of Public Health launch investigation into complaints of overcrowding at Pennhurst and growing population of feebleminded in Philadelphia and across Pennsylvania.

1913 Commonwealth investigation completed and report issued under signature of Dr. Joseph Neff, Philadelphia director of Public Health. Plans for further expansion at Pennhurst approved.

1919 Ten-year expansion program begins at Pennhurst, including Female Colony and a hospital.

1930 Despite economic depression, further expansion continues; male and female populations together exceed 1,500.

1936 Federal government and US Army Committee on Medical Research begin funding influenza vaccine and other trials at Pennhurst; medical experimentation will continue for three decades at Pennhurst and other institutions.

1957 Pennhurst population exceeds 3,500 residents.

1961 With addition of two annexes (Hamburg and White Haven State Schools) total population exceeds 4,100 residents; President Kennedy establishes White House Panel on Mental Retardation.

1968 In July, five-part NBC10 investigative report *Suffer the Little Children* exposes conditions at Pennhurst.

1971 On behalf of Arc of Pennsylvania, Thomas K. Gilhool and PILCOP file federal lawsuit claiming right to free public education for every child, including those at Pennhurst; 1972 consent decree lays groundwork for passage of 1975 Education for All Handicapped Children Act (now IDEA).

1974 *Halderman v. Pennhurst State School and Hospital* filed in federal court, challenging constitutionality of forced institutionalization and denial of services and protections in "least restrictive environment."

1977 *Halderman v. Pennhurst* trial in US District Court, Philadelphia. Judge Raymond Broderick rules in favor of Pennhurst class members (residents), declaring forced institutionalization unconstitutional. Court orders Commonwealth to devise strategy for community-based services. Multiple appeals follow, including two petitions to US Supreme Court.

1981 Six-year-long Pennhurst Longitudinal Study publishes first compelling evidence that majority of residents who have moved into the community "are better off," with greater quality of life than in institution.

1982 In *Romeo v. Youngberg*, Supreme Court overturns lower court and rules in favor of Nicholas Romeo in civil rights suit against the Commonwealth and Pennhurst; final settlement in 1984.

1985 District court approves Pennhurst Consent Decree, which affirms right to live in community and paves way for Pennhurst's closure.

1986 Portion of Pennhurst campus transferred to Department of Military and Veterans Affairs for veterans home; another area becomes National Guard headquarters.

1987 Pennhurst Center closes after almost eighty years of continuous operation; residents relocated to Community Living Arrangements (CLAs) (a few moved temporarily to other institutions).

1990 Americans with Disabilities Act (ADA) signed into law.

2008 Pennsylvania Department of General Services approves sale of property to Pennhurst Associates, Inc., for $2,000,000; Pennhurst Memorial and Preservation Alliance (advocacy group) formed.

2010 In April, Commonwealth Bureau of Historic Preservation erects historical marker to commemorate Pennhurst; Pennhurst Haunted Asylum attraction opens in October.

2018 In November Governor Tom Wolf signs SB 353 approving PMPA to purchase Superintendent's Mansion for a disability museum and interpretive center.

# *Suggestions for Further Reading*

There are few book-length studies that explore adequately the origin, history, and social policy consequences of a single institution dedicated to the confinement of individuals with intellectual and developmental disabilities. This volume seeks to address that deficiency while suggesting new avenues of scholarly research that have social and public policy significance. The study at hand raises larger questions about the nature of citizenship, equal protection under the law, the evolution of biomedical ethics, and the role of medical science in an age of professionalism.

This work rests on a foundation of primary and secondary research, oral interviews, and the personal recollections and experiences of individuals associated with the enduring struggle for disability civil rights. As the extensive endnotes indicate, there is a wealth of published and unpublished material, including archival collections, state government reports and pamphlets, memoirs, and websites. The list of sources below is not meant to be an exhaustive compendium; rather it offers accessible general works for readers who wish to read further on relevant topics bearing on the history and social context of Pennhurst State School and Hospital. The suggested readings complement the more specific endnotes. These are merely *suggested* readings and in no way exhaust the voluminous literature, nor supplant the materials found in the endnotes to this volume.

## ONLINE SOURCES


Asylum Project. http://www.asylumprojects.org/index.php/Main_Page.
Massive international research project on global history of institutions, organized by country of location.

Cold Spring Harbor Archives. http://library.cshl.edu/special-collections/eugenics.
Archives offer a compendium of manuscript holdings and projects sponsored by the Eugenics Research Office in the United States and abroad.

Disability History Museum. https://www.disabilitymuseum.org/dhm/index.html.
In addition to museum guide and other resources, site contains useful bibliography of printed and published sources in disability history.

Eugenics Archives (Canada). http://eugenicsarchive.ca.
Detailed website that contains a wealth of information—encyclopedia, timelines, teaching materials—on the eugenics movement in Canada.

Eugenics Archives (United States). http://www.eugenicsarchive.org/eugenics/list2.pl.
Contains the archives of the American eugenics movement, with extensive virtual exhibit and thousands of images illustrating range of the movement.

H-Disability. https://networks.h-net.org/h-disability.
Scholarly discussion forum that also contains book and article reviews, and other teaching resources.

Museum of disABILITY History. http://museumofdisability.org.
Online museum with very useful bibliography and teaching materials.

Pennhurst Memorial and Preservation Alliance Website. http://preservepennhurst.org/default.aspx?pg=6.
Richly detailed website and portal to the history of Pennhurst State School and Hospital, complete with timelines, bibliography, and other documents.

Vermont Eugenics Project. http://www.uvm.edu/~eugenics.
Monumental website devoted to the history of eugenics, with state-by-state detail of the impact of eugenics and institutionalization in the United States.

#### PENNHURST STATE SCHOOL AND HOSPITAL

Hornblum, Allen M, Judith L. Newman, and Gregory J Dober. *Against Their Will: The Secret History of Medical Experimentation on Children in Cold War America*. New York: Palgrave Macmillan, 2013.

Pirmann, J. Gregory, and the Pennhurst Memorial and Preservation Alliance. *Pennhurst State School and Hospital*. Images of America Series. Charleston: Arcadia, 2015.

#### DISABILITY HISTORY

Beckwith, Ruthie-Marie. *Disability Servitude: From Peonage to Poverty*. New York: Palgrave Macmillan, 2016.

Fleischer, Doris Zames, and Frieda Zames *The Disability Rights Movement: From Charity to Confrontation*. Philadelphia: Temple University Press, 2001.

Longmore, Paul K. *Why I Burned My Book and Other Essays on Disability*. Philadelphia: Temple University Press, 2003.

Longmore, Paul K., and Lauri Umansky, eds. *The New Disability History: American Perspectives*. New York: New York University Press, 2001.

Nielsen, Kim E. *A Disability History of the United States*. Boston: Beacon Press, 2012.

Pelka, Fred. *What Have We Done? An Oral History of the Disability Rights Movement*. Amherst: University of Massachusetts Press, 2012.

Rembis, Michael, Catherine J. Kudlick, and Kim E. Nielsen, eds. *The Oxford Handbook of Disability History*. New York: Oxford University Press, 2018.

Rose, Sarah F. *No Right to Be Idle: The Invention of Disability, 1840s–1930s*. Chapel Hill: University of North Carolina Press, 2017.

Schweik, Susan M. *The Ugly Laws: Disability in Public*. New York: New York University Press, 2018.

Trent, James. *Inventing the Feeble Mind: A History of Intellectual Disability in the United States*. Amherst: University of Massachusetts Press, 1994.

Wehmeyer, Michael L. *The Story of Intellectual Disability: An Evolution of Meaning, Understanding, and Public Perception*. Baltimore: Brookes, 2013.

Wolfensberger, Wolf. *The Origin and Nature of Our Institutional Models*. Syracuse: Human Policy Press, 1975.

## SCIENCE, POLICY, AND EUGENICS

Bashford, Alison, and Philippa Levine, eds. *Oxford Handbook of the History of Eugenics*. New York: Oxford University Press, 2012.

Begos, Kevin, Danielle Deaver, John Railey, and Scott Sexton. *Against Their Will: North Carolina's Sterilization Program and the Campaign for Reparations*. Apalachicola, Fla.: Gray Oak Books, 2012.

Black, Edwin. *War Against the Weak: Eugenics and America's Campaign to Create a Master Race*. New York: Four Walls / Eight Windows, 2003.

Bruinius, Harry. *Better for All the World: The Secret History of Forced Sterilization and America's Quest for Racial Purity*. New York: Alfred A. Knopf, 2006.

Cohen, Adam. *Imbeciles: The Supreme Court, American Eugenics, and the Sterilization of Carrie Buck*. New York: Penguin Press, 2016.

Degler, Carl N. *In Search of Human Nature: The Decline and Revival of Darwinism in American Social Thought*. New York: Oxford University Press, 1991.

Friedlander, Henry. *The Origins of Nazi Genocide: From Euthanasia to the Final Solution*. Chapel Hill: University of North Carolina Press, 1995.

Kevles, Daniel J. *In the Name of Eugenics: Genetics and the Uses of Human Heredity*. Cambridge: Harvard University Press, 1995.

Lederer, Susan E. *Subjected to Science: Human Experimentation in America Before the Second World War*. Baltimore: Johns Hopkins University Press, 1997.

Levine, Philippa. *Eugenics: A Very Short Introduction*. New York: Oxford University Press, 2017.

Lombardo, Paul A., ed. *A Century of Eugenics in America: From the Indiana Experiment to the Human Genome Era*. Bloomington: Indiana University Press, 2001.

———. *Three Generations, No Imbeciles: Eugenics, the Supreme Court, and* Buck v. Bell. Baltimore: Johns Hopkins University Press, 2008.

Maranto, Gina. *Quest for Perfection: The Drive to Breed Better Human Beings*. New York: Scribner, 1996.

Paul, Julius. "'Three Generations of Imbeciles Are Enough': State Eugenic Sterilization Laws in American Thought and Practice." PhD diss., Walter Reed Army Institute of Research, 1965. https://readingroom.law.gsu.edu/buckvbell/95.

Porter, Theodore M. *Genetics in the Madhouse: The Unknown History of Human Heredity*. Princeton: Princeton University Press, 2018.

Roberts, Dorothy. *Fatal Invention: How Science, Politics, and Big Business Re-Create Race in the Twenty-First Century*. New York: New Press, 2011.

Rosen, Christine. *Preaching Eugenics: Religious Leaders and the American Eugenics Movement*. New York: Oxford University Press, 2004.

Sheffer, Edith. *Asperger's Children: The Origins of Autism in Nazi Vienna*. New York: W. W. Norton, 2018.

Smith, Daniel J., and Michael L. Wehmeyer. *Good Blood/Bad Blood: Science, Nature, and the Myth of the Kallikaks*. Washington, D.C.: American Association on Intellectual and Developmental Disabilities, 2012.

Washington, Harriet A. *Medical Apartheid: The Dark History of Medical Experimentation on Black Americans from Colonial Times to the Present*. New York: Random House, 2006.

Zipf, Karin L. *Bad Girls at Samarcand: Sexuality and Sterilization in a Southern Juvenile Reformatory*. Baton Rouge: Louisiana State University Press, 2016.

# *Contributors*

**Dennis B. Downey**, PhD, is professor of history emeritus at Millersville University and a board member of the Pennhurst Memorial and Preservation Alliance. He is the author of numerous books, articles, and op/ed pieces, and has a special interest in American social thought, race relations, and the history of disabilities. The recipient of awards and citations for both his historical scholarship and disability advocacy, Downey served as president of the Pennsylvania Historical Association from 2005 to 2007.

**James W. Conroy**, PhD, has been a student of the disability rights movement for more than four decades. Since his first visit to a large public institution in 1970, he has committed his life to finding out how American society can do better than the shameful, inhumane conditions he saw. He has studied the well-being of people who have left institutions, including Pennhurst, in a dozen states, and is now working to extend what America has learned to the rest of the world. Conroy is CEO of the Center for Outcome Analysis and copresident of the Pennhurst Memorial and Preservation Alliance (PMPA).

**Ginny Thornburgh** is the former first lady of the Commonwealth of Pennsylvania and an internationally recognized disability rights advocate. She is an accomplished author, speaker, and advocate. Among her many contributions, Ginny Thornburgh served as director of Interfaith Initiatives for the American Association of People with Disabilities (AAPD).

**Richard "Dick" Thornburgh** is the former governor of the Commonwealth of Pennsylvania and subsequently served as United States attorney general from 1988 to 1991. A former federal prosecutor, he has long been active as a disability rights advocate. Thornburgh was attorney general at the time the Americans with Disabilities Act was enacted into law (1990).

**Janet Albert-Herman** is the mother of a young man with Down syndrome, and she has spent most of her career as an advocate/volunteer in the disability rights movement at the local and national level. She is one of the founding members of the Pennhurst Memorial and Preservation Alliance.

**Mark Friedman**, PhD, is adjunct associate professor of Disability Studies at the City University of New York (CUNY). He has worked on deinstitutionalization federal court cases in five states, supported self-advocacy organizations, and helped found the national self-advocacy organization, Self-Advocates Becoming Empowered.

**Nancy K. Nowell** is director of Social Signals, an organization founded to develop educational materials that teach safe relationships skills to adolescents and adults with intellectual disabilities and/or autism. She has been an advisor to Pennsylvania self-advocacy organizations for twenty years and worked for the federal district court overseeing the closure of Pennhurst.

**J. Gregory Pirmann** was employed at Pennhurst Center from 1969 until 1986, working as a caseworker, unit manager, special assistant to the superintendent, and as the director of Planning, Evaluation, and Development. He also worked at Embreeville Center and in the Southeast Regional Office of Developmental Programs before retiring in 2007. Pirmann is an officer of the PMPA and in 2015 published *Pennhurst State School and Hospital* (Arcadia).

**Bill Baldini** is the Philadelphia news reporter who produced the groundbreaking 1968 five-part series *Suffer the Little Children* that exposed conditions at Pennhurst. A watershed moment in expository journalism and disability rights, *Suffer the Little Children* raised public awareness of institutional conditions across America. Named "Newscaster of the Year" in 1998, upon his retirement in 2006, Bill was the longest-working television reporter in the city of Philadelphia. In 2005 the Philadelphia City Council declared March 17 "Bill Baldini Day," and two years later he was inducted into the Broadcast Pioneers of Philadelphia's Hall of Fame.

**Emily Smith Beitiks** received her PhD in 2011 in American Studies from the University of Minnesota. She now serves as associate director at the Paul K. Longmore Institute on Disability at San Francisco State University.

**Elizabeth Coppola** joined the Pennhurst Memorial and Preservation Alliance in 2009, where she served as secretary on the board of directors. In 2015, Elizabeth joined Purdue University and is pursuing her PhD in human development and family studies.

**Heath Hofmeister** is a writer and filmmaker with a commitment to disability rights, and is the writer and director of *A Call of Conscience: Pennhurst State School and Hospital* (2010). A graduate of the Millersville University School of Communication, he now lives and works in the greater New York metro area.

**Judith A. Gran**, Esq., is a partner in Reisman Carolla Gran LLP, a firm in Haddonfield, New Jersey, with a national practice in disability law. She represented the Arc of Pennsylvania and the plaintiff class in *Halderman v. Pennhurst* during the implementation phase of that litigation. She has represented institutional residents in cases that resulted in community inclusion and the creation of comprehensive community services systems in Oklahoma, New Mexico, Illinois, Montana, Tennessee, Connecticut, Delaware, and Pennsylvania.

**Nathaniel Guest**, Esq. is a graduate of Cornell University (BA, MA) and the Temple University School of Law (JD). A lecturer and specialist in historic preservation planning and law, he helped found the Preserve Pennhurst organization and the Pennhurst Memorial and Preservation Alliance. Guest is the recipient of numerous awards, including the Burton Award for Legal Achievement (2010) and the Temple University Friedman Prize for Legal Writing (2010).

**Chris Peecho Cadwalader** is the father of three children, two of whom have learning disabilities. A retired urban explorer, he became interested in Pennhurst at an early age. He created an informational website dedicated to Pennhurst's former residents to spread awareness of institutionalization in America. Together with Nathaniel Guest, he founded the Pennhurst Memorial and Preservation Alliance (PMPA).

# Index